Victory Over Your Big Fat Body

by Mike Shane, ESP
elementary school pupil (1950)
Moshe4442003@yahoo.com

with Wes Bagby, genius
friend
wes0007@hotmail.com

Printed in the United States of America

This book contains the opinions and ideas of its author. It is sold with the understanding that the author and publisher are not engaged in rendering medical, health, or any other kind of professional health care advice. The reader should consult a qualified health care professional before adopting any of the suggestions in this book.

The author and publisher disclaim all responsibility for any liability, loss, or risk, personal or otherwise, which is incurred as a consequence, directly or indirectly, of the use and application of any of the content contained in this book.

ISBN: 978-0-9844664-0-5

Library of Congress Control Number: 2010901634

Contents

Contents

Acknowledgments

This is dedicated to the following wonderful people who were kind enough to help me, or teach me, or love me, or heal me enough to make the book happen: Grandma Gussie, Dr. Stanley Chaing, Susan Shane, Ibrahim Sola, Donna Bronson, Rose Marie Venuto, Dr. Ernest Vargas, Wen Chau, Joel Perlish, Miss Mullen, Wes Bagby, Dr. Steven Shane, Tom Shane, Dr. Dean Ornish, Joshua Reinstein, Izik Shahar, Lorie & Jake Kopenhaver.

May you all be blessed forever by a Spirit of Loving Kindness.

Miracle

An unexpected event, often thought of a perceptible interruption in the laws of nature. A wonderful, unlikely beneficial happening believed caused by a higher power, or a miracle "worker."

Angel Of Death

THE ANGEL OF DEATH IS A CONCEPT THAT HAS EXISTED SINCE THE beginning of history. In English speaking nations he is known as the grim reaper. Grandpa Fink called him "Uncle Jerry" and feared him mightily, as does the author of this book.

In some cases, Uncle Jerry is able to actually cause death, leading to stories of ways to bribe or trick or outwit him in order to extend one's life. Jerry's job is to escort the deceased to the after life.

Behavior
Modification

BEHAVIORISM IS BASED ON THE PROPOSITION THAT JUST ABOUT everything we do (feelings, thinking, acting) should be regarded as behavior.

Business uses this "science" to "hook us" into buying their products time after time. Many of these "products" are harmful to our waistlines and health.

"Good" behavioral guidelines in this book show you how to escape from the "bad," addictive, harmful, poisonous garbage that is peddled out there to us and our children.

"Good" behavioral science can help us create new, improved lifestyles with better health, more vigor, more happiness, and less weight.

Paranormal

Outside the range of normal experience or scientific explanation.

The scientific community generally does not support what is characterized as the paranormal. But over half of Americans believe in psychic/spiritual healing. We are agnostic about science, except when it hurts us. Believing in the paranormal approach to life is lots more fun.

I.

Path to a Miracle, Part 1

A<small>T AGE</small> 65, I <small>WAS LIVING IN THE VALLEY OF THE</small> S<small>HADOW OF</small> D<small>EATH.</small> Cancers and heart disease depressed many of the folks who lived along Sanibel Way in Bradenton, Florida, me included. Our fears competed with noisy parties as to what would dominate the neighborhood on any given day.

The bus that Uncle Jerry (Angel of Death) drives picked up two neighbors in July 2005. I knew Jerry was driving up my driveway too when I felt the fading breath/sounds of a dying man, me.

> *Death is one appointment we must keep,*
> *but for which no time is set.*
> —Charlie Chan

Coughing was continual. I couldn't sleep. My heart raced to an irregular and rapid rhythm. Breaths were shallow and got weaker amidst fits of coughing. My chest was sore, achy, and hurt a lot. The cough alone taught me what it's like to dance with death. Intimate as hell, but no fun. Moving beyond the toilet ten feet away became too long of a trip.

"Shane, see a doctor," demanded a son, a girlfriend, and a wise Latino nurse from across the street who made me chicken soup.

After a month of misery, I saw the doctor. In his view, I was a medical mess; congestive heart failure, enlarged heart, atrial fibrillation, and blood pressure so high it was out-of-sight. He said I was close to being worse off than dead. Worse than dead? Hmm, how could THAT be?

When you stroke out, he explained, "it can be. Listen Shane, go to the hospital. You've got serious problems. I'll send over specialists to treat you."

If this is dying, I don't think much of it.
—Lytton Strachey

I didn't go to the hospital. A few weeks later the stroke arrived as predicted. It caught my attention enough to consult with a cardiac/stroke specialist in Sarasota. He wanted to operate the next day. It would be a "minor" procedure that would normalize my heartbeat. After that, he wanted me to take eight heart/stroke pills a day for the rest of my life. These included Warfarin™, a blood thinner also used to poison rats.

When my favorite neighborhood nurse told me about the rat killer, I snatched back control of my medical destiny from the physician(s). I turned down the surgery and six of the eight pills he wanted me to take. "Shane, take the Warfarin. It's what you need."

I don't believe in miracles—I depend on them.
—Raymond Dale

If my health gets screwed up even worse, I said, let it be all my fault. It's my body. Live, die, or lingering in a situation worse than death can't be worse (to me) than swallowing poison.

> *Have the courage to live. Anyone can die.*
> —Robert Cody

The second stroke came two months later. My left arm wouldn't move, scratch, lift, grasp, push the TV remote, nothing. Feeling was gone. The arm was indifferent to the rest of me. It hung down, dead.

The third stroke happened in April 2006 and this event wasn't a cause for celebration either. My ability to speak was replaced with the babbling sounds of an eight month old. Nor could I read, write, or walk normally. My once brisk walking gait was replaced by a slow, sluggish limp.

Uncle Jerry was closing in again. The short list for bus pick up surely included me. For no reason that I remember, I wanted to live longer. I wanted a "just not now" delay on death. I decided to cash my social security check and, like a kid, just run away. Perhaps I'd try to retire in reverse, to the north. I'd hide somewhere away from Uncle Jerry and those medical experts who offered to treat my medical condition with rat poison.

> *Death is a very dull, dreary affair and my advice to you*
> *is to have nothing to do with it.*
> —Somerset Maugham

(Find MIRACLE again in last part of book.)

II.

How to Lose Weight
(behavioral change section)

YOU ARE READING THIS BOOK BECAUSE YOU'RE FAT AND YOU NEED to lose that excess weight. You want to become more attractive, have more energy, live healthier longer, and even improve your sex life. Less weight on you offers those opportunities and costs much less than remaining overweight. Eating addictive and toxic foods, or even too much food with high nutritional value, will kill you too soon. Overeat and even your own heart may attack you.

Holiday feasts make large numbers of us drop dead. Fear holiday dinners no longer! Help is here—finally—and it's in this book!

If being nonfat brings better health, more joy in life, more energy, why get fat in the first place? We didn't put in for that.

REASONS WE ARE FAT:

- We love to eat fattening, salty, addictive foods.
- We eat too much. We can't stop when we should. Our stomach and cravings say "more" and we obey. Our brain has been hijacked and is sick.
- We never heard of healthful foods while growing up.
- We crave the satisfaction of "comfort foods".
- We believe that tracking HOW we eat takes too much time.
- Healthful eating tips have been irrelevant to us.
- We believe that obesity runs in our family.

> *People say that losing weight is no walk in the park.*
> *When I hear that I think, yeah, that's the problem.*
> —Chris Adams

We prefer foods loaded with tasty but toxic chemical concoctions, foods that make us fat, then sick, then prematurely dead in 15 or 20 years. Geniuses out there successfully market addictive foods (CAN you stop after just one salted potato chip?). We stood little chance against creamy, sugary, salty, chewy, and deadly foods—until now.

The good news: Helpful behavioral and nutritional suggestions in this book will show how our shopping habits can be changed so the harmful foods sold at the grocery store are ignored and never make it to your kitchen. You will soon shop the right way to lose the weight that you want. Your fix on fattening foods will end, and you will get thinner.

> *I'm not overweight. I'm just nine inches too short.*
> —Shelley Winters

This victory also could eliminate disease: diabetes, digestive tract disorders, cardiac conditions (broken hearts?), strokes, and much misery.

Dad's massive stroke happened at 68. He had high blood pressure. He routinely enjoyed bacon, French fries, pork chops, pastrami (ribs anyone?). Tragic endings like Dad's are predictable when harmful foods are your favorite foods.

> *As for food, half of my friends have dug their*
> *graves with their teeth.*
> —Chauncey M. Depew

It's a simple truth: Harmful foods are killers just like cigarettes. Your choice: Live longer via mindful, healthful dining, or walk around in a fat body and die sooner and sicker by continuing to do what you've been doing. Any education we have received about food has been pathetic. Job #1 is to learn a lot more about the stuff you swallow (that becomes YOU). Sensible ways to make our bellies flat and bodies lean are out there, and we need to learn about them. This book will show us exactly HOW to become thinner, healthier, happier, and remain so (see healthful food choices listed in food section).

If millions of smokers can learn to quit a difficult tobacco addiction, and they have, we can learn how to quit addictive foods.

Statistics don't lie (unless liars compile them). No foreign nation ever killed more Americans than the honorable folks out there who sell us harmful foods/beverages, tobacco, and legal drugs.

> *If food is your best friend, it's also your worst enemy.*
> —Grandpa Jones (1978)

But hey, the good news is soon you will learn how to walk away from fattening foods because this book teaches you how. You will actually prefer healthful foods over harmful foods, and you won't need to overeat to be full. You will get thinner, healthier nearly every day until you reach your optimum weight.

FAT FIGHTING AT ITS BEST:

Start a blog
Get a dog
Take a class
Move your ass
Don't just talk, walk the walk.
Cut harmful additives and sugar
for natural fruits and a veggie burger.
Bad food has made you fat.
Good food will bring you back.
Wrong food has made you depressed
Right food will make you feel your best.
Blessed with new positive energy
You can exercise and become happy
So throw out the cupcakes and Twinkies™
And ride a bike while you watch TV.

—Wes Bagby

Choosing healthful foods helps a lot, but alas it's not enough to get the job done. As the poem noted, to reach your best weight, you need to do more than simply eat less. You also need to move about much more. "Move your body" isn't just a musical refrain, but an absolute essential to losing weight. From now on, move briskly around your home, outside, even at work (if it won't get you fired). Stand, don't sit in front of your TV. Stretch, twist, swing arms, lift legs, do yoga posturing or participate in the 6 a.m. TV exercise show. Be a couch potato no longer. Better yet, turn the damn TV off and go outside for a walk. While you're becoming more active, unglue yourself from the computer (my intention after this is written).

—*Simple Math*—

Sensible portions of healthful food + movin' about often,
vigorously = a slimmer, healthier you.

Mindless eating habits got you into this mess. Becoming mindful will bring you out of it. Until now, you missed out on life's good stuff: a leaner body, optimal health, plenty of energy. Right now, making two simple changes can turn the next two weeks of the rest of your life into very important ones.

Eating less bad food, and moving about with energy and vigor will remind you how good it feels to live healthfully. Your body, your mind, and your heart will thank you.

You have decided to love and take care of yourself and the wonderful thing you will find is that your mind and your body will start returning the favor and start loving and taking care of you in return. Welcome to the first phase of your recovery and your freedom.

> *We stand at a fork in the road.*
> —unknown

LOSE 5 POUNDS IN 14 DAYS

> *In any diet, the first thing you'll lose is your temper.*
> —unknown

Speedy Weight Loss Menu

BREAKFAST 6 to 9 a.m. (after a brisk 2+ mile walk)
One large apple, or pear, or orange, or eight plump purple/red grapes, + half a ripe banana. Eat your fruity breakfast slowly.

Coffee? Take it black and w/o sweetener.
Or herbal tea. . . . Good without adding sugar.
A multiple vitamin probably can't hurt.
Drinking more water will make you feel fuller.

LUNCH 11 a.m.–2 p.m.
Choose:
Veggie egg white omelet, tossed salad (fat free dressing), 9 unsalted nuts, piece of fruit, herbal tea or water, half a sweet potato

or

4 to 6 oz. chicken parts★, green veggie (baby spinach, etc.), 10 unsalted nuts, half a sweet potato, piece of fruit, herbal tea.

   ★Bake an hour at 400 degrees. Remove skin and enjoy.

DINNER 4 to 6 p.m.
Choose:

Cherries Jubilee (mix 10 frozen cherries with scoop of low fat yogurt). Top with slices of leftover banana from breakfast

or

Bowl of Shredded Wheat with Rice Dream or 1% milk.
Top with sensible number of raisins and/or blueberries.
Add the banana left-over.

   Much less food and far more exercise will reduce your weight noticeably in two weeks. You'll wonder where that weight went, but don't worry, you won't miss it. You'll feel good, with more energy. Weigh yourself now and again in two weeks. Show your stuff. Improve your diet. Impress yourself.

Dieting is not a piece of cake.
—unknown

BECOMING THINNER STEP BY STEP

Brisk walks tighten your stomach, curb your appetite, and burn calories. If you walk about a mile per day now, add 3 or 4 miles daily (around an hour) of BRISK walking. Being with a friend (or almost anyone) makes a long walk seem shorter, more pleasant. To lose the weight you want, there's no time not to walk. Strolling won't get the job done since it doesn't burn enough calories. Also, a fast walking pace will carry you further from your refrigerator, another good thing.

10

No diet should be an on-again, off-again affair. If all you do is go on it until you lose some weight, then go off it, chances are you're among the 90% of all dieters who will regain the weight they lost soon after leaving their diets.

To make your weight loss permanent, something more than a diet is needed; rather a new way of eating. You need to change HOW you eat, not only what you eat. The habit changes suggested in this book will help you adopt a healthful diet that can be permanent. This does not mean you can't eat your favorite food any more. It does mean you need to control or reduce the size of portions, your snacking, and learn the reasons why you overeat, then correct them.

> *All the things I really like to do are either*
> *immoral, illegal, or fattening.*
> —Alexander Woollcott

The book is based on scientific principles developed by experts in a field called behavior modification. Using "B Mod", people have been able to kick smoking addiction, overcome mental issues, and yes, lose weight permanently. The techniques can be learned and applied easily in the privacy of your home. You won't need a personal counselor, just the ability to monitor your own behavior and follow instructions.

The first important step is to get a clear picture of what, how much, and under what conditions, you eat and overeat. You will need to keep a personal food diary for awhile.

> *If you fail to plan, you plan to fail.*
> —proverb

Happily, to lose weight safely, you won't need to stick to celery, or grapefruit, or water, or just a few food items to lose weight. You can prepare hundreds of tasty dishes that will help result in less of you.

You will get thinner by following the step-by-step instructions that follow. You need a weight loss goal. How many pounds do you want to lose? Let's say it's 30 pounds (your goal may differ). Then your job is to lose 1–2 pounds a week methodically, logically, safely until you achieve your goal.

No need to starve or get very hungry, even if you decide to go on a modified (fruit, water) fast. More on this later. When you get to your right weight, better eating habits will kick in to keep you there. You will have learned how to control your weight and better weight control means better life control.

I think I just ate my willpower.
—unknown

IN THE BEGINNING. . .

For a week (or longer), keep a journal. To lose weight and keep it off, accurate records are important. No one likes it, but what you put on paper during your transformation to a slimmer self will be helpful in many ways.

You can gain control over your eating behavior and keep it under control by creating daily menus at least one day in advance for a set number of meals: 2 or 3 main meals, and 1 or 2 small snacks such as an apple, evenly spaced throughout the day. Be sure to include more water in the mix. Then remain strictly loyal to your own menus. After dinner, write down what you intend to eat the next day. Find good ideas in the food section.

Design menus with the goal of slim and healthy in mind. Foods selected should be nutritious and not leave you craving additional food. When you are satisfied with your menu list and portion sizes, resolve that what is on the list will be the ONLY food you allow yourself. Make menus for the next month. After that time you can recycle your menus with slight variations.

Stay away from junk foods such as sugared or diet sodas, cookies, doughnuts, chips, French fries, hot dogs, etc. Keep them out of your house. For "snacks" that pick you up, fresh fruits, raisins, carrots, or some unsalted nuts are your best bet.

If it's too much to prepare a new meal daily, then prepare larger portions and enjoy them tomorrow and the next day. Create your healthy menus when you are NOT hungry.

Include all the items you intend to eat and drink, the time, and the portion size. Eat normally, but from now on, stay away from the addictive, fattening, salty, sugary foods listed in the food section.

> *I'm in shape. Round is a shape, isn't it?*
> —unknown

After a week of record keeping, evaluate what you ate and drank. Did you eat too much at a certain time of day? What about portion size? Any after dinner raids on the fridge or cupboard? Any binges? Any relapse to "bad foods"? Now the menus will help you control this tendency.

Menus consisting of healthful foods and planned by you a day or a week in advance will help control overeating. And be sure to end all eating at 6 p.m. Night-time eaters weigh about 8% more than day time eaters even when both groups eat the same amounts of the same foods, according to researchers. They don't know why.

Make adjustments downward if portion size concerns you. But if your stomach growls, it may initially need to contract a bit to get used to reduced portions. Later, if still hungry, add foods with more protein such as hummus, fish, hard boiled egg whites, skinless baked chicken, etc. to the menus. Don't allow your growling stomach to trick you into gluttony or binge eating.

In any clash of wills, your mind should prevail over your stomach. Positive awareness will produce healthful eating. More pleasure will come from eating less food less often. Remember, the hungrier we are, the better the taste of our food.

> *The vilest of beasts is your belly.*
> —Greek proverb

Note any unusual aspect of your eating in your journal. Do you snack when tired, bored, or angry? Do you have a "worst" snack time? As you review the past week, consider what caused you to eat and overeat. Journaling identifies what bad foods went into you, when, and why.

Move about vigorously. Find stairs and climb them. Instead of driving, walk briskly. Spend less money on gasoline and more on walking shoes. Exercise at home, at the gym, anywhere.

Lose weight sensibly. Don't try to break any records. A pound or two a week will take you to your weight destination quickly enough and safely. Weigh yourself weekly about the same time of day and record it. Less weight this week than last will make you feel better about yourself. More weight, or being stuck too long on a "plateau", means you need to revisit your diet strategy and make changes. Dieters who weigh themselves periodically lose more weight than those who don't. The scale seems to motivate dieters to take immediate steps, such as decreasing portions or exercising more when their weight plateaus.

Important Behavioral Suggestions:

- EAT SLOWLY. It is important that you take your time because your stomach needs 20 minutes to tell your brain it has taken in enough food and is full. Put your fork down between bites to help you slow down.

- DRINK water before meals. It helps fill us up, and lots of times when we "feel" hungry, we are simply thirsty. Maintaining an attractive body isn't easy, otherwise nearly all of us would be slender and look terrific. Thin folks tend to keep fattening foods out of the house. Some fast on Tuesday, weigh themselves Wednesday, then celebrate via vigorous gardening on Saturdays. What it takes to be thin is what they do. Fat folks don't work nearly as hard as skinny ones, or live as long.

> *Take care that your hearts are not weighed*
> *down by overindulgence.*
> —Luke 21:34

TECHNIQUES OF SUCCESSFUL DIETERS

- KEEP OUT of the house what's not on the approved food list. Why be tempted?

- DEFEND against snack attacks. Determine vulnerable time(s). Plan strategy with a friend.

- DRINK more water. (To successful dieters, this one was most helpful.) Drinking lots of water made them feel fuller.

- BE MINDFUL of what's on your plate before it goes into you.

- Smaller plates make it seem like you're eating more.

- Take your meals at the same place, at the same time.

- ENJOY breakfast. Even if just toast and tea, don't skip breakfast.

- Occasionally, nonfood rewards are helpful to good dieters.

- GIVE away non-fitting clothes.

> *Don't dig your grave with a knife and a fork.*
> —proverb

Still More Suggestions

- DON'T STARVE yourself or allow long periods of time to pass without eating something healthful.

- NIBBLE at raw veggies before meals to take the edge off your appetite.

- FIND A DIET BUDDY. Losing weight with someone helps a lot. Successful dieters have the support of family and/or friend(s). Try to find a relative or friend to participate with you.

- READ FOOD LABELS. Avoid foods that add salt, sugar, & artificial anything. They can be addictive. Pass on prepackaged lunch meats. They aren't good for you. Fresh is always best.
- CREATE daily menus several days in advance and stick with them.

> *Let food be your medicine.*
> —Hippocrates

REWARDS

As you know from reading this far, success at dieting is no easy task. If it were, there would be fewer failures among dieters who definitely want to, but can't lose weight and keep it off. Already you know enough proper eating habits to lose weight, but will you practice them from now on? Perhaps, but. . . .

Most of us perform better, diet-wise and otherwise, when we know there is some reward for a job well done, not only when the goal is finally achieved, but occasionally along the way. To help you succeed where others have failed, consider making a reward system part of your weight loss program. Here's what we mean . . .

- Take a few moments to be proud of yourself each day that you remain faithful to sensible menus. Congratulate yourself, pat yourself on the back. You deserve it. The fact that you are becoming a slimmer, more attractive person should motivate you to maintain a "thin" diet.

- Note how much better and healthier you feel while getting closer to your desired appearance and optimum weight. Think of the pleasant activities in life you will enjoy more once you get thinner. So reward yourself frequently with happy thoughts while making progress, AND after you get there.

- Provide visible rewards for maintaining good eating habits. For example, give yourself a "check mark" for every day you keep your diet. Log the checks in a notebook only on days you shun harmful foods and don't overeat. Leave blanks for the days that you relapsed.

Upon earning checks for seven consecutive days of good eating practices, exchange them for an inexpensive personal gift—but something you value: a movie, a favorite magazine, etc. Have a good time. You deserve it. Or, if you are a delayed reward type of person, save the check marks for a month, then lavish some attention on yourself, something that feels good and is healthful (a nice massage, a pair of warm gloves, a new book, a weekend night at a nice hotel with your significant other, etc.).

Good news! Even your favorite (bad) food can become a useful part of your reward strategy. Let's say you love Rocky Road ice cream. You cannot imagine continuing a food journey through life without it. Well cheer up. You may enjoy a sensibly sized scoop of Rocky Road as part of your reward system, but only away from home. Obtain your favorite food in reasonable portions as a reward for maintaining good dietary practices for at least two weeks. If a treat like ice cream helps keep you on the right food track, it can be a good thing.

> *My advice if you insist on slimming: Eat as much*
> *as you like, just don't swallow it.*
> —Harry Secombe

To help maintain your dietary routine, continue the reward system for six months. By then your eating habits will be turned around to "slim" and you will prefer them to your former practices. Looking at the new you in the mirror every day will be reward enough.

> *When hungry I eat, when tired I sleep. Fools laugh at me.*
> *The wise understand.*
> —Zen Master Rinzai

SOLUTIONS TO WEIGHTY PROBLEMS

The Problem
I stopped losing with 24 pounds to go.

Solutions

- For one week, take another inventory—meticulous and truthful—of your eating habits.

- Remove foods from your house that cause excessive weight gain.

- Create new "thin and healthy" menus and follow them.

- Prepare smaller portions! Eat slowly. Chew more.

- Reward yourself with praise and a cup of coffee or tea for every "thin" meal you eat.

- Become more attentive to the behavioral suggestions.

- Walk more, watch TV less.

- Leave a bite or so of each food on your plate. Do this and it gets easier to stop eating, even before you're "full". Being full may mean that you've already eaten too much. Get used to walking away from the table without feeling obligated to empty your plate.

- A "modified" fast once or twice a week may be your ace in the hole. It's a sure-fire way to lose weight. More on fasting later.

The Problem
I binge twice a week. Am I a loser?

Solutions

- NO, forgive yourself and quickly climb back on the diet wagon with new determination. There's good reason to believe this will not be a future problem. Binges become less frequent when more nutritious meals are prepared.

- If possible, keep those foods that make you binge out of the house. Or keep them in small enough quantities that binging on them is impossible. Make fruit and raw veggies the most abundant and accessible items in your fridge. Don't leave sugared or salted high calorie leftovers around. They often are too tempting to resist another urge to binge. Become kitchen savvy. Get smarter than the folks who sell food that makes you eat too much.

- Several drops of olive oil on half a bagel, eaten slowly, can turn off hunger. So will a ripe banana.

- Next time you feel a binge coming on, reach first for cool water or a container of low sodium vegetable juice. Pour a large glassful, sip it, relax, feel thin, and trust that the urge to binge soon will fade away.

- Get out of the house more. Join a dance group that meets after work (when many binges happen). Returning home very tired after a gym workout makes it unlikely you'll think about food. Like fasting, exercise can actually curb appetites.

- YOGA will provide the willpower to defeat binging. Learn it. Besides improving your body's flexibility and strength, yoga can make you smart about food. Those who practice yoga are tuned into their bodies and appetites. They are good judges of how much they actually need to eat and are capable of walking away from food still on the plate. Yoga requires focus and paying attention to one's body. It will help train you to eat less, and not binge.

> *The devil came to me last night and asked what I wanted*
> *in exchange for my soul. I still can't believe*
> *I said pizza. Friggin' cravings.*
> —Marc Ostroff

The Problem
My family isn't supportive. Is it dumb to diet?

Solutions
- Explain how successful you intend to be, and invite one of them to join you. Say how much it would mean if you had their blessings.

- Emphasize how beneficial your permanent new eating habits are; how a better diet helps to avoid heart disease, stroke, diabetes, varicose veins, and other ailments.

- If no support is forthcoming, change the subject when talk turns to your diet.

- Maintain current relationships but make new friends. Join a diet group with members who will be supportive to you. Dieting together with someone is more effective than dieting alone.

> *You better cut the pizza in four pieces because*
> *I'm not hungry enough to eat six.*
> —Yogi Berra

The Problem
ANGER makes me overeat.

Solutions
- Turn to humor to cool your anger. Laugh at a funny movie or comedy on TV. Buy a funny book (like this one). Try to find a funny side to almost all situations. Think of doing something hilarious, then do it.

- Remember that white breads, pasta, and other starchy stuff may turn you into a depressed or angry person. Stay away from foods made with white flour and replace them with fruit and veggies, plus drink more water.

- Learn yoga. Meditate. Walk a mile in the fresh air. All can diffuse anger.

The Problem
I get TIRED, then eat too much.

Solutions
- Go to bed and count each breath you take. Fall asleep fast from boredom and dream of becoming thinner and more

attractive. Enjoying enough sleep may actually keep your body from storing fat. Lack of sleep increases cravings for fattening foods like ice cream and pizza and a triple cheeseburger.

- Shrug off fatigue and engage in some vigorous sex. You'll burn calories and it will take your mind off food for awhile. When you're finished, get up, wash up, sip some tea, and take a walk.
- Take a hot shower (or cold one) if someone has a headache.

> *Be plain in dress, and sober in your diet. In short,*
> *my dreary, kiss me, and be quiet.*
> —Mary Worley Montegu

The Problem
GLUTTONY

> *Gluttony is an emotional escape, a sign something is eating us.*
> —Peter de Vries

Solutions

- Drink low or no calorie beverages 20 minutes before meals (water, low salt veggie juice, unsweetened tea, etc.).
- Chew your food slowly and thoroughly. Put the fork down between bites. Those who eat quickly and until they are full are three times more likely to be overweight than those who eat slowly and leave the table before getting full.
- It's important to reduce the size of food portions. Portion control is one of the most important ways to defeat obesity, but it's hard to do for many dieters. It'll take a conscious effort and a big change in how we think about food.
- Think thin from now on. Take the view that any food piled high (even when nutritious) is the major problem of the moment, and one that needs your immediate attention. Did you recently cave and buy a chocolate cake? Gift it quickly to a thinner neighbor without eating any of it. Unhealthful foods

quickly need to be placed out of sight and out of reach of fork and spoon. Vow that the foods at your next meal will reflect your diet goal.

- Use a salad plate instead of a dinner plate at mealtime. It'll seem like there's more food in front of you. Eat "thin" foods, vegetables and high protein foods like hummus, almonds, and low-fat cottage cheese. Less harm will occur from occasional overeating if you consistently reduce your portion size.

> *Tell me what you eat, & I will tell you what you are.*
> —Antheime Brillat-Savarin

- BECOME MINDFUL about your eating behavior. Pay attention to the food in front of you; its taste, the pace of your chewing, swallowing, even consider whether your body is getting ENOUGH nutritional stuff. Become totally aware of the eating, not what's happening in the living room. Concentrating on your meal means you will likely eat less. Postpone discussing various topics until you're finished eating.
- After a few weeks of mindful eating, you will begin to control overeating rather than it controlling you. Focus on the food in front of you. Allow your mind, not your stomach, to guide you through lunch and dinner.

> *It's not what you're eating, it's what's eating you.*
> —unknown

The Problem
I'm LONELY, so I overeat.

Solutions
- Join a group whose members engage regularly in activities you enjoy. Is there an Overeaters Anonymous or Weight Watchers group near you? Does the local gym sponsor diet classes?

- Volunteering will take you out of the house to where you can display your generous nature. Love animals? Shelter dogs would wag tails when you show up. What about your local library? Plenty of exercise stacking all those books. Become a big brother or big sister and soon you'll become a big hero to a small child.

- Learn something new like painting, music, belly dancing, magic, floral arranging, gardening, sports, cooking healthfully. Then seek out others who share your interest.

The Problem
STRESS makes me overeat.

Solutions
- Exercise is a great stress reducer. Do more swimming, biking, gardening, and hiking. Exercise your mind with hobbies like painting or bird watching; Scrabble™ or puzzles.

- Meditate and learn yoga. Either one can calm you down without spiking your appetite.

- Enjoy beautiful music, make new friends, play with kids.

- Visit the comedy channel where humor easily trumps stress.

- Avoid foods containing processed sugar. They can cause mental issues AND obesity. (More cake?)

> *Why is 'desserts' spelled backwards 'stressed'?*
> —unknown

FASTING YOUR WAY TO THINNESS

Many diet winners fast weekly to become and stay thin, especially those holding sedentary jobs. Within that group, some enjoy fasting so much they increase it from once a week to every fourth or fifth day.

> *Fasting is the best medicine.*
> —Indian proverb

Our "modified" fast begins at 6 p.m. and lasts for 36 hours. Drink lots of water throughout the fast. Twice a day, when you're at your hungriest, enjoy modest amounts of fruit, 6–8 grapes or cherries, or an apple, or half a banana, etc. Fruit will provide that food boost you need to pacify a growling stomach. Your body will let you know when the fruit is most appreciated.

Expect to lose a pound or more per fast. You'll probably feel less hungry after the fast than before it began, another good thing. Fasting curbs appetites but like other behavioral change suggestions, it is not an on-again, off-again tool. People who fast weekly should do so the rest of their lives. Those who "go off" their fasting generally regain the weight they lost.

Fasting is considered one of nature's best healers. When ill, animals stop eating instinctively. People who fast report more energy, more health, more vitality.

> *Dieters live life in the fasting lane.*
> —unknown

Lose Weight, Get Paid

Dieters who "get paid" for losing weight lose about three times more weight than those who don't. And here's where there is a big benefit to belonging to a weight loss group.

An inexpensive, competitive way to lose weight and win money is to bet on your success. Here's how: Six (or 8 or 10) members of the group agree to compete with each other for a month. They place $10 (it could be more) into a collective jackpot at the beginning of the month. The biggest losers of weight in the next 30 days become jackpot winner(s). It's that simple.

All participants weigh in at the same time on the same scale. A month later, they weigh again on the same scale at the same time. The top two in weight loss share the money, $30 each, surely enough to make you much more aware and mindful of proper eating practices during the month. If you don't win the first month, too bad. Simply try harder next month. Lose more weight and you will be a winner, one way or the other. Meanwhile, fun competition among dieters can be rewarding!

> *If you wish to grow thinner, diminish your dinner.*
> —H.S. Leigh

III.

Curbing Your Appetite

(The Food Section)

- *SUPERSTAR foods—21 Winners*
- *SANITY foods*
- *MEMORY foods*
- *NEGATIVE CALORIE foods*
- *HEART HEALTHY foods*
- *BELLY FAT fighting foods*
- *MIXED BLESSING foods*
- *MINDFULNESS vs. mindlessness*
- *COFFEE AND TEA, good for thee! Not so fast*

- *EAT MORE SUGAR for more cancer*
- *MORE SALT for more strokes*
- *BRAIN HIJACKING foods fatten your butt & belly, then kill you*
- FOOD TITANS: *supersize the greedy jerks*
- WORLD'S OLDEST MAN—*how he did it*

APPETITE CURBS

Ever wonder if certain foods could fill you up in the morning and keep you satisfied pretty much the whole day? Well wonder no more; a terrific weight loss breakthrough has arrived via the research of diet and obesity expert, Dr. Louis Arrone, MD. He has identified foods that make and keep you full; healthful, high protein foods that along with colorful veggies provide the nourishment you need, and eliminate those hunger pangs.

Curbing your appetite in the p.m. is all about eating foods high in protein in the a.m. Here are some suggestions:

Appetite Curbing BREAKFAST Ideas—
Veggie EGG WHITE Omelet: (top choice)

- rye toast, coffee or tea or water
- piece of fruit
- no butter, cheese or hash brown potatoes

This is a tasty meal AND an effective appetite suppressor.

> *There is no such thing as a pretty good omelet.*
> —French proverb

- TUNA or salmon sandwich: rye toast, mustard, lettuce, tomato, etc.; applesauce on the side. Coffee or tea. (good for lunch too)

- PEANUT BUTTER on rye with pure fruit spread. Hot tea plus an apple. You'll feel like a happy kid again.
- OATMEAL with low fat vanilla yogurt, raisins or berries, a dollop of maple syrup. Cool days become warm. Better yet, do oatmeal for dinner!
- SLICED BANANA atop 1%, no-salt-added (Friendship) cottage cheese, with coffee or tea, rye toast. Quick, easy, healthful.
- FRUIT SHAKE—Blend lots of frozen blueberries, spoonfuls of vanilla low-fat yogurt, a banana, some skim milk. Great anytime.

OTHER morning ideas to rein in later day cravings:

- baked chicken (remove skin before eating);
- hummus and cucumber on low salt or no salt crackers;
- poached salmon with spinach & apple slices.

WHY RYE?

Rye is a grain bread that fills you up and also keeps your hunger at bay for many hours. Researchers found that two slices of rye toast in the morning will decrease hunger both before and after lunch. But do not buy "rye" bread that's not really rye. Most breads sold as "rye" contain more wheat than rye. Make sure rye is the MAIN grain in the loaf. Read food labels. The food industry is not always honest with what they call their foods. Buy only real rye bread!

LUNCHES THAT CONTROL CRAVINGS

Let a healthful, tasty salad END your lunch to better nudge the other foods through your digestive system. Baked fish from cold waters should be your lunch guest (salmon, tuna, halibut, haddock, mackerel, etc.) to prevent overeating later in the day. If you prefer sushi, it is delicious, filling, healthful, but expensive. Chicken is relatively cheap and can be baked easily. Hummus, cottage cheese, and beans/legumes are good protein foods. Add spinach, yams, and other colorful veggies for a nourishing, low fat meal. Fry nothing, except egg whites. Even here, boiling a hard boiled egg is the healthier option. Boil, broil, bake, poach, grill your way to weight loss.

Hunger is the best sauce.
—proverb

VITAMINS & FOOD CRAVINGS

A vitamin/mineral supplement containing calcium and vitamin D could reduce your cravings for certain foods. In one study, female dieters ate less fatty food and lost much more weight than women who didn't use this supplement. Their bodies no longer "craved" fatty foods that contain calcium (ice cream). Vitamin D helps a body better absorb the calcium.

Take a daily vitamin. There could be something useful to your body there that it hasn't been getting, and will add to your overall health. It costs little and makes some sense.

LIGHT DINNERS & SOUPS

Soup's on! Delicious, inexpensive, low calorie, highly satisfying, easy to prepare—soup should be a favorite food of healthful dieters who are determined to lose weight and keep it off. Load your soups with vegetables that will fill you up and make you feel good. For more heft in your soup, microwave a cut-up sweet potato and toss it into the pot. Nothing beats a clear chicken or vegetable broth soup made from scratch and flavored with sage, thyme, pepper, etc. Dessert? Cherries jubilee (pitted cherries in low fat vanilla yogurt) will make you cheer. Unless you forgot your apple, eating should end around 6 p.m.

> *My doctor told me to stop having intimate dinners for four*
> *unless there are three other people.*
> —Orson Welles

IMPORTANT BEHAVIORAL TIP: Shop for food when you are full! If you shop on an empty stomach, you'll be much more likely to buy foods that made you fat in the first place. Shop after you have eaten, or when you are not hungry. This will make it easier to select the right foods and avoid the wrong ones.

SUPERSTAR FOODS—21 WINNERS!

Healthful foods have enormous healing power, in contrast to junk foods' evil power to seriously undermine your health. Here are 20 superstar foods that will help make you thin. A few are previewed in some detail to show how incredibly wonderful they work inside of you.

Apples

Apples are seriously healthy and you should become a dear food friend to them. To help curb your appetite, enjoy an apple before a meal. The fiber in it expands in your stomach to help you feel full longer.

Apples are low in salt, and one consumed per day may well keep doctors at bay. They don't add water weight to your body mass. They are low in calories, and contain a source of dietary fiber that draws bad cholesterol out of us. They are cancer fighters. Can any producer of salty, sugary peanut butter cups say that? An apple also delivers antioxidants to fight cancer of the prostate and lungs. This fruit may also help slow the aging process.

How about apples and weight loss? High in fiber but low in calories, apples fill you up but not out. Enjoy apple wedges before meals to give your weight loss efforts a boost. Wash but don't peel an apple. The peel has anticancer properties and protects our body cells.

Beans & Lentils

Lentils, first cousin of the bean and pea, are among the most healthful foods. Served alongside veggies (tomatoes, peppers, broccoli, onions, garlic, etc.), lentils are protein rich, nutritious, and cheap. Think lentil stew and that's a lot of what you need to know about healthful dieting.

In 2008, the "Mediterranean" menu was considered by many to be the most healthful in the world. Lentils are the centerpiece of the menu. They help protect your heart; their fiber lowers cholesterol and keeps blood sugar levels from skyrocketing. And with lentils inside you, your bile will flow smoothly. Kidney beans, peas, and black beans are some foods in this group.

Egg Whites

Great protein source, few calories, and low in fat. They fill you up and curb your appetite. Buy the egg whites in a carton or hard boil several eggs and allow your dog to lap up the yolks.

Fish

Alaskan fish (salmon, halibut, etc.) are caught in less polluted waters than other ocean or river fish, but are more expensive. Low in calories, high in protein, three or more servings per week of fish will make you healthier and thinner than eating the flesh of a land animal.

Hummus & Seitan

Arabs and Israelis agree at least on one thing. Hummus is tasty and good for you. This bean-based, high protein food goes well with sliced cucumber on a low salt cracker or in a flat bread tomato sandwich. It can take the place of mayonnaise. Or enjoy hummus any way you care to imagine. Seitan tastes great and is a good protein source. You can make seitan chicken stew or seitan sausage that tastes like a beef stick. Check it out for healthful salads or however you like.

> *BEHAVIORAL TIP: Slow eaters tend to weigh less than rapid ones. Fast eaters are likely to be overeaters. Slow down!*

Nuts
These dry oily seeds are favored by squirrels and people for their good taste and high nutritive value. Keep your nuts free of salt to avoid becoming addicted to them. Limit the nuts near your plate to about ten. They are loaded with calories. On a positive note, folks who favor nuts eat less junk food and live 2 to 3 years longer than those who don't.

Grapes
Grapes, raisins, and red wine are fighters of cancer and heart disease. Purple concord grapes will sharpen your mind. Grapes and wine are featured in the Bible, so that's good enough for me.

Cauliflower
Eaten cooked, raw, or pickled, cauliflower is nutritious, high in fiber, low in fat, and a cancer fighter. An excellent substitute for starchy potatoes and a first cousin to healthful, green broccoli.

> *I'm President of the United States and I'm not*
> *going to eat any broccoli.*
> —George Bush, Sr.

SOUPS, STEWS, VEGGIE CHILI
Soup equals a hundred different healthful food blessings. Low in cost, few in calories; buy soups, stews, and chili that say "low salt"

on the container. Better yet, drop a colorful array of veggies into a pot and cook up something more delicious than you thought possible. Enjoy soups for supper. You will lose weight.

Shredded Wheat

Shredded wheat helps us move our bowels. Try some bite sized shredded wheat before taking any bowel movement problem to a lower authority. The fiber in this cereal pushes every other food through your digestive pipes fast, and that can also have a cleansing effect. Also, if you feel an evening binge coming on, mix shredded wheat, rice milk, blueberries, raisins, and bananas in a bowl and go for it (if you absolutely must).

Spinach

Vitamin rich spinach gave Popeye his power and his good looks. Because of spinach, Popeye didn't suffer from macular degeneration or obesity.

> *If it grows out of the ground or someone can pick it*
> *off a tree, chances are it's good for you.*
> —Unknown

Cottage Cheese

High in protein and simple to use, this tasty dairy food will fill you up and keep you satisfied for a long time. Goes well in the a.m. with rye toast, pure fruit spread, and tea. Eat low or no fat cottage cheese and yogurt products to help you lose belly fat.

Blueberries

Blueberries are a powerhouse food all by themselves, or atop cottage cheese, yogurt, in a fruit shake, etc. They reduce blood pressure by thinning blood (in contrast to salt). They help reduce age-related diseases and long-term memory loss. There's more too, but I forget.

Vegetable Juice

Drink a glass of low or sodium-free veggie juice before lunch or dinner. It will curb your appetite and improve your health, a win-win way to lose weight. Mix in some purple grape juice to improve its taste.

Tomatoes

What's a sandwich without some slices, or pizza without a tomato-based sauce, or a salad without its orange/reddish color? Tomatoes are a daily "must" food item. They fight cancer and heart disease. Another good thing is you can chase away war mongers and politicians with the single toss of a rotten tomato, making them feel so unwelcome that they leave.

Bananas

Many humans and chimpanzees believe bananas are nature's perfect food. This yellow fruit may lower high blood pressure and protect us against heart disease. Caution: Bananas are high in calories. Limit yourself to one or two medium-size bananas a day.

> *The belly is ungrateful. It always forgets we already gave it something.*
> —proverb

Sweet Potatoes / Yams

Sweet potatoes have one of the highest nutritional values of all vegetables, a veritable warehouse of vitamins and fiber. Yet Americans eat only about four pounds a year of this great food. That's down from 31 pounds in 1920. No shock that cancers have prospered in some correlation to the decline in the quality of our food choices. We supersize the addictive junk food, but decrease consumption of our super foods, like yams.

Oatmeal

Big health benefits from oatmeal when enjoyed as part of a low fat eating lifestyle. It lowers cholesterol and the risk of heart disease. It fills you up before you overeat. It tastes great with yogurt, cinnamon, raisins, blueberries, honey, or maple syrup.

Cabbage

An excellent source of fiber and vitamins, cabbage has great taste cooked or raw as in coleslaw. Stuffed cabbage can make a delightful meal. Cabbage soup can heal the coldest soul. To the ancient Greeks and Romans, cabbage surpassed all other vegetables.

Rice and Soy Milk

We prefer rice or soy milk over animal milk. Something just seems strange about human grown-ups drinking the milk of a four-footed creature. Give me vanilla rice milk with shredded wheat and lots of blueberries swimming in it.

Avocados

Avocados contain vitamins and minerals that promote good health. Slice them into salads or float some on soups. They replace butter, mayonnaise, and cream cheese in sandwiches or atop bagels. They add protein and flavor to your meals. However, an avocado contains more calories than just about all other plants, so enjoy them sparingly.

Additional FRUIT Winners:

- Cherries, Berries, Plums, Mango, Dates,
- Figs, Oranges, Prunes, Cantaloupe, Honeydew,
- Strawberries, Watermelon, Peaches, Pears.

Healthful Favorite Veggies:

- Asparagus, Cucumber, Broccoli, Peppers, Eggplant,
- Collard Greens, Brussels Sprouts, Garlic, Mushrooms,
- Pumpkin, Beets, Celery, Zucchini, Lettuce, Onions, Carrots.

> *Sex is good, but not as good as fresh, sweet corn.*
> —Garrison Keillar

Sanity Foods

Eating certain fish (especially wild salmon and mackerel) can help keep us sane. The risk of dementia and cognitive function (forgetfulness, confusion, memory loss) drops when fish is eaten by seniors 2–3 times a week. Replace red meat, believed to help cause dementia, with healthful, cold water ocean fish.

Walnuts aren't called "brain food" for nothing. They look like a brain. And this nut produces better cognitive functioning and brings us heart healthy benefits. Nutty as this sounds, walnuts also may make you thinner.

Foods for Mental Nimbleness

MUSTARD—Turmeric in mustard activates genes that clean up our brains.

EGGS—Selenium in eggs fights aging in the brain.

BLUEBERRIES—Compounds in this berry slow down brain aging and are a good alternative to sugar snacks (blueberries in vanilla yogurt, yum!).

SPINACH/kale/collard greens—These leafy heroes slow mental decline.

PEPPERMINT TEA helps you focus and boosts mental performance. Drivers become more alert and are less anxious after a cup of mint tea.

NUTS & YOGURT help you calm down in stressful situations. Add half a cup of wheat germ to your yogurt or oatmeal to increase physical endurance and your body's ability to deal with stress.

MEDITERRANEAN MENTAL HEALTH

The Mediterranean Diet concentrates on small portions of high quality foods and has been linked to better mental health. This diet is rich in veggies, fish, nuts, fruits, lentils, and grains. Olive oil replaces butter and margarine.

One study found that the Mediterranean diet is superior to a high cereal, high fiber diet when it comes to certain risk factors for heart disease and lowering blood sugar (important to diabetics). Northern Europeans and Americans eat more meat, potatoes, and fattening deserts than Italians and Greeks, and suffer more obesity.

> *Much meat—much disease.*
> —Proverb

NEGATIVE CALORIE FOODS

Some fruits and vegetables burn more calories in the digestion process than they contain. Carry this absurdity forward if you can, and accept the notion that the more of these foods you eat, the more weight you may lose: They include apples—asparagus—beets—broccoli—cabbage—carrots—cauliflower—celery—cucumbers—grapefruit—lettuce—oranges—pineapples—raspberries—spinach—strawberries—turnips—zucchini.

> *This cabbage, these potatoes, these carrots, these onions*
> *will soon become me. Such a tasty fact!*
> —Mike Garofalo

STIFLE STARCHY FOOD

Replace starchy foods—white bread, white potatoes, white rice—with healthier, more nutritious high roughage foods like multigrain breads, sweet potatoes, and brown rice. Better nutrition means you will probably need to eat less. Thus you will weigh less.

BELLY FAT FIGHTING FOODS

Foods containing flavonoids can reduce our belly bulge by increasing body metabolism. Here are some examples: pears, apples, tea, very dark chocolate, onions, beans, sweet peppers.

HEART HEALTHY FOODS

GRAINS—rye bread, oatmeal, low fat/low sodium whole grain breakfast cereals.

VEGGIES—asparagus, Brussels sprouts, broccoli, artichokes, cabbage, squash, carrots, greens, green beans, peas, pumpkin, mushrooms, onions, spinach.

> *An onion can make people cry, but there has never been a veggie invented to make them laugh.*
> —Will Rogers

> *Second Opinion: Do not eat garlic or onions for their smell will reveal that you are a peasant.*
> —Cervantes

FRUIT—plums, tomatoes, apricots, berries, raisins, prunes, pineapples, melons, peaches, mangoes, oranges, grapes, cherries, dates, applies, figs, bananas, pears, strawberries.

FISH—herring, sardines, salmon, mackerel, other finned fish caught in cold ocean waters and not raised on fish "farms". Salmon served in most restaurants comes from a "farm" and is inferior.

LEGUMES etc.—lentils, unsalted nuts, beans, peas.

OILS—olive, safflower, canola, fat free cooking spray.

ACID AND ALKALINE FOODS

Go easy on foods that turn acidic in your body. Too much acid may weaken your bones and muscles. Eating alkaline foods produces the opposite effect.

ALKALINE foods: Nearly all fruits and veggies.

ACID-forming foods: alcohol, bread, beef, cereal, milk, pork, cheese, eggs, nuts, rice, sausage, chicken, pasta, cow's milk, potatoes.

MIXED BLESSING FOODS

NUTS—Healthful and nutritious, nuts are addictive when salted and have a ton of calories. Dieters should set a limit on numbers BEFORE each nutty experience. Do we need all the salt and those disabling, deadly strokes that come of it?

> *To eat is a necessity, to eat intelligently is an art.*
> —la Rochefoucauld

DARK CHOCOLATE—A delicious food that could lessen the damage from heart attacks (buy dark chocolate with at least 60% cacao). Want to be smarter and pass your next test? Small portions of dark chocolate increase cerebral blood flow. But here's the negative catch. Chocolate makes us fatter and spawns chocoholics. Sugars, fats, and salt in chocolate are unfriendly to dieters. Also remember to clean your teeth promptly and properly after each chocolate experience to help avoid a $1,600 root canal. Shun milk chocolate altogether. There are no health benefit and lots of nutritional downsides.

OIL—Although a few are healthful, oils are fattening. Use it in moderation on salads and pizza and about everything else for flavor enhancement. Canola and olive oil are much more heart friendly than oils from beef, pork, and chicken, but just as fattening. To lose weight, use LESS oil than previously. For example, prepare your own healthful salad dressing (yogurt & cucumber pieces is one healthful example). Buy non-salty, low calorie commercial salad dressings.

CHICKEN—Before eating, remove the skin and fat to eliminate much of the bad stuff. Buy chickens that aren't pumped up with hormones, additives, water, etc. Read the labels. Bake chicken parts in a pot that contains a grill so the fats can drip out during the cooking process. Don't fry chicken.

BREAD—Whole grain breads are OK in moderation if you don't add fats to them (butter, margarine, cream cheese). Breads made with white flour are a pathetic excuse for food and contain lots of salt and empty calories. They spike your appetite, making it likely you'll overeat later on.

> *Never eat more than you can lift.*
> —Miss Piggy

SIZE DOES MATTER

If there's no measuring cup, use your fist to determine portion size for the main items of your meal. Just about every portion should be about the size of your fist.

GROCERY STORE FAVORITES

- COTTAGE CHEESE—Friendship brand is our favorite. Buy the container with 1% fat, "no salt added" clearly printed on the label. Great taste, but be careful. It's easy to buy a salted Friendship cottage cheese by mistake.

- PEANUT BUTTER—Crazy Eddie's™! Love his name & his product. Imagine, a peanut butter containing just one item, peanuts! Joseph's™ Crunchy Valencia peanut butter and Whole Foods™ brand are other good picks.

- MARINARA SAUCE—Trader Giotto's (Joe's)—no salt added, low fat. Search diligently. The salt free jar was almost hiding amidst hundreds of other salted sauces sold by Joe. Bake a delicious pizza at home using this sauce, low fat cheese, wheat flat bread, mushrooms, etc. Tastes just as good as "regular" pizza and isn't harmful to your health.

- HUMMUS—The Sabra™ brand and Sonny & Joe's™ are especially delicious. Great for sandwiches and other stuff. Lots of healthful protein.

- CRACKERS—Triscuit's™ "Hint of Salt" is a tasty, crunchy cracker. Finally a giant food company bakes something that's fun to chew and helps you go. Low in fat, low in salt, low in cholesterol. High in satisfaction.

- FRUIT SPREADS—Several companies sell healthful, spreadable fruits. These can replace jellies and jams that are loaded with processed sugar.
- TABATCHNICK™ LOW SODIUM frozen soups—Great tasting, great family name. Look for their blue packages. They contain soups with less salt and say so on the label. An excellent source of protein and fiber, low salt soups are better for you than pizza or pasta or virtually any food that begins with the letter "p".

> *One cannot think well, love well, sleep*
> *well if one has not dined well.*
> —Virginia Woolf

MINDFULNESS vs. MINDLESSNESS

Do you taste your food before swallowing it? I mean really taste it—for flavor, for chewiness, for freshness, for fun. Or is mealtime simply a quick food inhaling experience while your mind trips over your work, your money situation, your family? If that's the case, you're missing out on how proper eating can help you lose weight and lead a healthier, freer, more joyful life. Food has been controlling you, and it needs to be the other way around.

Allow the pathway to better health and lower weight to take shape through positive thinking. We need to be keenly aware and focused on what is allowed to enter our bodies. Being mindful (mindfulness) is how it's done.

Little else in our lives, except sex perhaps, is as intimate as the eating of food. When we don't focus like a laser on food in all its aspects—purchase, preparation, consumption—it becomes a mistake that results in poor food choices and fat people. Not focusing on food helps make people obese in the first place. Remaining mindless about your meals and snacks (just shoveling food into you without enough thought) means you will remain overweight, and die too soon.

When you focus on why you buy certain foods, how you prepare them, and when and how much you eat, you enable yourself to lose weight.

What caused your weight to go out of control? One reason is you have not related to food in a mindful manner. If you had, you'd never have allowed eating to become a curse when it should be a blessing. You buy and eat harmful comfort foods without thought. You eat too much, too fast, and too frequently that you don't consider the consequences. It's time to put your eating behavior under your own control. Don't leave control of how you eat to fate, or some giant food company that peddles sweet, salty, addictive, fattening crap.

Why should clever TV ads and "irresistible" foods conspire with our "mindlessness" to bring us harm? Is Coke™ really it? Doesn't NOBODY not like Sara Lee™? Why eat any foods that can cause your brain to misfire?

> *Strength is the ability to break a chocolate bar into four pieces*
> *with your bare hands—and then eat just one of those pieces.*
> —Judith Viorst

Unless we become mindful of our eating, food producers, not us, will determine how many years we remain on this lovely planet. Companies will sell whatever addictive stuff they can get away with. They will try their best to get us to buy what we "need" for the rest of our fatter, briefer lives. (Need sugar and cream in your coffee?)

Folks, be mindful of what goes into you. Shop when you're NOT hungry. Think a bit before you buy the bad stuff; you may change your mind. Becoming mindful about your food matters. It will help you lose those bulges in your body. Mindfulness can empower us to achieve a thinner, healthier life. It can defeat food addictions and prevent harmful, fattening foods from entering our bodies.

Focusing on foods and snacks is not easy. You need to consciously retrain your mind to serve the best interests of your entire body. Your thoughts mustn't be allowed to wander from the task at hand. When they do, nudge them gently back into focus. Consider food preparation (the merits of baking vs. frying). Mind how food smells, how it tastes, its texture, its origin, its cleanliness. Consider how it will make you feel in a few hours.

The right foods and you need to become good friends and that's a lot to chew on. But try to chew on it mindfully from now on.

Count the number of your bites per food item. How does chewing "feel" for you? Often the colors of natural foods relate to their nutritional value. Usually, the brighter the healthier. Think berries. Think green, leafy spinach. Consider the sweetness of a sweet (orange) potato. Inhale the aromas, not the foods. Enjoy your foods. Eat them slowly.

What's the mood around the table? Are those next to you as nice as you are? Or is there drama that's not doing you, the dieter, any good? Expand your senses as they relate to food. Look at food in some new ways. Eat as little as you like, not as much as you want. This is about you getting control over (finally)—you.

Perhaps most important to mindful eating is some display of appreciation of your connection to food and foods' connection to nature. Before meals, offer thanks for the gift of healthful food. Perhaps a silent prayer or a moment of meditation, or simply silence depending on your belief, or lack thereof. If you say a prayerful word or two about thy food, put in a good word for me (it can't hurt).

A mindful person forbids her/his stomach from making major food buying decisions at the grocery. One's mind, not the belly, should determine how much gets eaten at supper time. Your brain needs to become the decider, not the marketing department of some food company. Fend off corporate and stomach demands for you to eat salty, sugary, and fatty foods. Why allow a chronically irrational part of you (belly) to dominate how much you eat, how you look, and how sick you get? Mindful people use their minds to empower themselves to avoid harmful foods. They KNOW when enough food really is enough. They just get up, walk away, and leave leftovers for tomorrow.

> *Gluttony kills more than the sword.*
> —unknown

WHERE'S THE BEEF?

He was 70+ and the owner of a meat company that shipped perfectly aged sirloins and T-bones across the nation to restaurants and individuals. From personal experience, the sirloins were superb. I preferred his company's beef to all others. But when this prince of sirloin accepted our dinner invitation, we served salmon. I shared my negative health news with our successful visitor.

"Fish is fine." His response was quick and sincere. "We eat fish, and we like it, but I could never let a day go by without some meat on the table, and I have as much energy as I ever have—especially since they put in the heart stents" (surgically implanted devices that open up obstructed coronary arteries).

Hey, selling steaks is what this guy did for a living. Selling cigarettes is the job of the tobacco guys. Protecting ourselves from these guys' products has to be our responsibility. Who else?

The sirloin man loved selling steaks and was good at it for over 35 years. But the steaks that made him rich even broke HIS heart, and continues to break the hearts of countless steak "lovers".

To be sure, this book is not about the national medical crisis but the point is that ravaging our bodies with dangerous foods has serious national health consequences.

> *We have met the enemy . . . and he is us.*
> —Pogo

RULES OF EATING

Relax, simplify your food selections by following these rules of eating and you may not suffer diseases that come from eating perhaps the world's unhealthiest diet—the one offered by high tech food companies to you and me. Here's how:

- Don't buy foods that contain more than four or five ingredients. If a food company needs to jack its products with chemicals you can't pronounce, it's not (good) for you.

- If it don't rot, it should not be bought. Imagine the damage foods that are kept chemically "fresh" for weeks and months can do once they enter your gut, liver, heart, and brain. Don't bring rotgut foods home anymore. Eat mostly plants, bought fresh or frozen.

- Eat at specific times of the day. Enjoy meals with people you care about. It's a time for bonding with family or friends who enjoy being together.

- Stick with food favored by your great-grandparents. The 1900 generation didn't suffer epidemics that ravage 2010 America— diabetes, cancer, heart disease, obesity. Eat far less meat and select foods that contain no added salts or sugars.

> *Things sweet to the taste prove in digestion, sour.*
> —Shakespeare

- Try to limit the foods on your plate to three items or fewer at a time.

> *We eat less when less food is in front of us.*
> —anon

- Share dessert. You'll capture the flavor and miss half the calories.

- End your eating BEFORE you're full. Practice leaving the table feeling a little hungry. You'll burst with energy, and lose more weight.

> *When diet is wrong, medicine is of no use. When diet*
> *is correct, medicine is of no need.*
> —Proverb

COFFEE & TEA (good for thee . . . not so fast)

COFFEE UPSIDE: It's a disease fighter; it's a stimulant; it changes moods.

People who drink coffee weigh less than those who don't. It has no calories, but to lose weight you need to abandon, or at least strictly limit the creamy, sugary stuff most people "take" (a little skim milk can't hurt). If you don't, coffee becomes calorie rich and will help keep you fat.

Whether coffee is a dieter's delight or downfall is debatable. We're talking about a powerful food that may do you lots of good when used properly, but also can cause harm.

Health benefits of coffee include lowering the risk of diabetes and Parkinson's disease. Caffeine in coffee stimulates the brain and provides energy for longer exercise workouts or walks. Coffee speeds metabolism even while not exercising. Thus you burn calories and you lose weight. The beverage could even improve a sour mood. Taken around a table, coffee may make folks more receptive to each other's point of view. Those are the positives. Now for the flip side.

COFFEE DOWNSIDE: IT'S A STIMULANT. IT'S ADDICTIVE. IT CHANGES MOODS.

While appetites may be suppressed in the short run, many coffee drinkers' craving for food increases during the course of a day. The caffeine in coffee is an addictive drug that can manipulate your feelings downward as well as upward. That can't be good for your brain, or for your health.

> *Why does man kill? He kills for food. And not only*
> *food—frequently there must be a beverage.*
> —Woody Allen

47

If you wonder whether you are addicted to coffee, just try getting through the next two or three days without drinking it. You'll have proof soon enough. If you don't want to remain a coffee addict, cut back slowly. Because it changes your mood, coffee probably also interferes with your weight loss objectives.

Caffeine in coffee is a powerful stimulant that can prevent you from knowing which foods work well for you, and which ones don't. When caffeine represses your thought patterns and attitudes, it also may mask the effects of your eating. You won't know where your energy comes from, the food or the coffee.

A mindful eater and a coffee addict probably can't live comfortably in the same body. Coffee makes you feel wired, nervous, and edgy at times when "calm" might be better. Dieters should avoid caffeine in the morning. A cup after lunch may be OK, but take your coffee as Europeans do, with some water, making it easier on your stomach. Or simply take tea, and see. . . .

> *Only Irish coffee provides in a single glass all four essential food groups: alcohol, caffeine, sugar, and fat.*
> —Woody Allen

TEA: *The Dieter's Friend*

GREEN TEA is the most healthful of the tea beverages and dieters can feel good about drinking up to three cups per day. It contains no calories and only about half the caffeine of a cup of coffee. Ounce for ounce, few if any foods or beverages contain as many health benefits as green tea.

> *There is no trouble so great or so grave that cannot be diminished by a nice cup of tea.*
> —Bernard Heroux

Studies of tea and weight loss have been promising. Early conclusion: Oxidants in green tea reduce body fat and help control obesity. Besides caffeine, green tea contains substances that cause our bodies to burn more fat than would be eliminated by the consumption of caffeine alone. Green tea also helps us exercise longer, producing even more weight loss.

There is little downside to drinking green tea. It's not considered addictive like coffee though there's enough caffeine in a cup of tea to cause insomnia if taken too close to bedtime (try decaf then).

The good news about green tea is its growing reputation as a disease fighter. A powerful antioxidant in green tea, called EGOG, fights cancer, arthritis, heart problems, infection, and impaired immunity. Therefore if you intend to lose weight AND create a more healthful lifestyle for yourself, safe, nonaddicting, green tea is for you. It's an enemy of disease, and a destroyer of fat. Drink green tea straight, without sugar or cream. Drink it often.

> *Sour, sweet, bitter, pungent—all must be tasted.*
> —Chinese proverb

ADDICTIVE ADDITIVES

Let's face it, food makes us happy, reduces stress and gives us a temporary sense of satisfaction and comfort. Some of us have become a little too happy and have seen the results on our overly joyful waistlines. Food is an essential necessity of life—why shouldn't it make us happy? But could certain food neurons be firing in our brain in a dreadfully misguided way? Could food companies be inflating our joy of eating by addicting us to hike profits? Is there somebody behind the scenes inserting powerful ingredients into our food supply to make us feel that enough is never really enough?

Some facts follow that could scare you, but they also will help you take control of yourself from those food companies that are more concerned with profit margins than public health.

Ever wonder why our food cravings are never for broiled chicken, steamed broccoli, fresh fish, or fruit? Isn't it strange that food cravings always seem to involve foods that deliver the most calories, the most fat, the most sugar, and the most artificially induced taste into our bloodstreams? Pizza, chocolate, nachos, and ice cream find their way into our thoughts far too often. So why DO we think of these foods more than, say, Alaskan halibut?

I know what you're thinking: The answer is simple—because they taste good. And you're right. But let's ask ourselves why these foods taste so good that we reach for them over and over again rather than the more healthful, natural foods?

When we think about it, the almost amazing fact is that the closer a particular food is to its natural state, the less likely it is that we will have an unnatural craving for it. Since we know that fighting cravings is crucial to weight-loss success, this is valuable knowledge.

Processed foods that cause weight problems have been carefully engineered by food companies. They make us heavier, more depressed, and dependent on the same comfort foods we crave to fight the depression it caused in the first place. And, as an extra unwelcome bonus, they drain our energy to do anything about it.

We know what a vicious cycle this is from firsthand experience. And we know that the key to our success at becoming thinner lies in finding a way out of our artificially induced prison of emotionally driven eating. We must recognize a fearful fact: Food is a drug, and we are addicts. We buy drugs legally from the grocery stores, but our food addictions are not really any different from heroin, alcohol, tobacco, etc. They lead us to make food the central focus of our lives.

To break free, we have to understand why certain foods act as a drug in our bodies. Then we need to detoxify our way back to healthier eating. We must know what addictive agents are in our foods and how we can avoid them.

There are over 3,000 approved food additives in America. Almost all packaged foods contain some of them. They are essentially chemicals that change the natural properties of our food, and most are designed to make food look and taste better.

Preservatives are additives that keep bacteria from growing on our food, but they also enhance a food company's ability to increase the shelf life of its product. Here are some common and worrisome food additives.

ARTIFICIAL SWEETENERS: You might be surprised that NutraSweet (Equal, Aspartame, etc.) is found in 5,000 different food products, including some sugared ones. It's also found in 600 different medicines, including many children's medicines. Other artificial sweeteners include Sweet-n-Low™ , Splenda™, Tagatose™, and Neotame™. Studies have found that these artificial sweeteners actually have the effect of making you crave more calories than if you had eaten real sugar in the first place. It turns out that when you eat something sweet but do not take in any calories, your body reacts by increasing its cravings for the sugar calories that it missed.

In the long run, artificial sweeteners are just a marketing gimmick. They give you the short-term satisfaction of having sweets without the guilt, but the long-term effect is to keep you buying more to satisfy ever-growing cravings.

Those who use artificial sweeteners as a sugar replacement end up eating more of the specific item than if the item had real sugar. It's a win–win situation for the food manufacturers.

Artificial sweeteners have been widely used as food additives for nearly 20 years. America's weight problems as a nation has never been greater than for the last 20 years. There are concerns that using these additives produce bad health effects from long-term use. Studies point toward an addictive quality in artificial sweeteners. In fact, one popular product loaded with artificial sweeteners, diet soda, has a support group for "diet soda addicts".

Among other things, the group offers tips on how to detoxify from a diet cola addiction.

SUGAR HELPS CANCERS GROW

Refined sugar has many names (dextrose, glucose, fructose, maltose, corn syrup, etc.) and is present in nearly all processed foods. The average American consumes almost 200 pounds of sugar per year, about a half-cup every day. Sugar additives are insidious and their consumption increases in proportion to our weight problems. One study discovered 76 ways excessive sugar damages our long-term health. This is especially worrisome since nearly every American qualifies as an excessive sugar consumer. Apart from the one effect we all know too well—making us fatter—other effects include increased fatigue, arthritis, migraines, lower immune system functioning, gallstones, gum disease/cavities, heart disease, and many others. And recently, it was found that cancer cells inside our body prefer consuming sugar for their own maintenance and growth. How sweet is that?

Another study found that sugar is more addictive than cocaine. Lab rats already addicted to cocaine chose sugar when given a choice between the two substances. We know that controlling our sugar intake is essential to successful weight loss.

Of all the food additives, sugar is our most difficult challenge and easily the major reason why dieters fail to lose weight permanently. Not only does it taste good and is so easily available, but we are addicted to a substance that is considered as addictive as any we know of.

However, here's some good news. The treatment and cure for this addiction comes from an old friend: Mother Nature. Eating the natural foods suggested in this book is the quickest way to detoxify our body from the sugar "drug". Natural foods will restore our bodies to a more balanced metabolism and slowly decrease our cravings. And we will be blessed with energy and improved mental health.

HALT THE SALT

If nothing else in this book helps you out, please heed this warning about salt. It has become, and is, a major killer (about 92,000 Americans in 2008), and uncountable others are affected more indirectly. Salt contributes to high blood pressure/strokes, heart disease, kidney disease, and fluid retention. Reducing the amount of salt you eat will reduce your blood pressure and risk of a stroke. It will extend your life.

On the average, we eat about three times the amount of salt we should every day, and that excessive amount will screw you up badly before a stroke kills you. Here's what the Center for Disease Control said: "There is no room for debate any longer that a high level of salt causes stroke and heart disease, and that lowering salt intake will diminish these very serious health consequences."

Most excessive salt we eat comes from processed foods such as tomato sauce, soups, condiments, canned foods, and just about everything else you find on grocery shelves, even bread. Only a small fraction comes from the salt you add to food at home. It is vitally important that you check food labels so you can prevent yourself from buying foods with added salt (or MSG or baking soda).

What's a food company's chief executive to do? He doesn't WANT to kill you, but he NEEDS to keep you eating his company's products, good and bad, to keep his job. Being an effectively addictive agent, salt is loaded into foods to keep you coming back for more, no other reason. Is there a real difference between the makers of salty crackers and those who sell us cigarettes? Addicting shoppers is a great way for big business to make big bucks. Too bad millions will die too soon so food companies can profit so much. But, hey, that's life in the land of the free. (If you have some, light up now.)

Here's a ray of hope. Our taste for salt can change very fast. Food served with much less salt starts to become tasty after a couple of days. Besides avoiding harmful salty foods, here's what do to extend your life and become healthier.

- Compare food labels to find sodium free options.
- Look for foods containing no added salt, soy sauces, etc.
- Be smart. Use herbs and spices to replace salt. Seasoning blends such as Mrs. Dash contain over a dozen tasty herbs and spices that will help you to lose your salt craving fast.
- Replace salt with flavored vinegar.
- Use sodium free or low sodium chicken broth.
- Eat more fruits and veggies. They are naturally low in sodium.
- Before eating them, RINSE and drain foods that are usually loaded with salt. These include pickles, olives, canned vegetables, canned tuna, etc.

SODIUM NITRATES

These preservatives are added to foods such as bacon, corned beef, ham, lunch meats, sausage, pepperoni, and, of course, hot dogs. They are used to prevent the growth of bacteria and give meat a falsely healthful-looking pink color. Nitrates are considered dangerous by the FDA, but they haven't been banned largely due to their ability to prevent spoilage and botulism.

The World Cancer Research Fund reports that adults and children who consume processed meat risk developing cancer. The American Institute for Cancer Research has recommended not just limiting consumption of processed meats but that we avoid them completely due to overwhelming links to cancer.

This should concern us. Statistics show Americans eat 20 billion hot dogs a year. This is about 70 hot dogs per person on average. Researchers note that just one ounce of processed meat a day hikes our risk of stomach cancer up to 38 percent.

MSG™ (MONOSODIUM GLUTAMATE)

What's the first thing that you think of when you hear MSG? If it is "Chinese food," then this section should be a real eye opener. MSG is a flavor-boosting additive that is found in nearly all processed foods and in nearly all fast food restaurants. It has become one of the key tools used in the arsenal of the food manufacturers to enhance flavors and to get you addicted to their food.

And, as we will discover, just because the food label doesn't mention MSG by name, it doesn't mean much. There are other names that can be legally used. For example, are you aware that when a food label mentions "natural flavorings" or "spices", these are legal terms for MSG?

The Japanese had been adding seaweed extract into their food for thousands of years because it enhanced flavors. In the early 1900s, an enterprising Japanese researcher isolated the flavor-enhancing chemical compound, MSG, within the seaweed extract. Two years later, the first food additive company to produce MSG was created. This Japanese company was named "Ajinomoto" which roughly translated means "essence of taste". Today, Ajinomoto is a multi-billion dollar food additive company, and the world's largest producer of MSG.

In the late 1960s, a neuroscientist began studying the effects of MSG on mice in his lab and discovered that it caused health issues and obesity. MSG is referred to as an "exitotoxin" because it kills brain cells by "exciting" them to death.

The effects of MSG were discovered to have especially concentrated effects on young mice. Alarm was raised and the food industry was pressured to voluntarily agree to remove MSG from baby food. However, even at this day, this agreement remains purely voluntary and the FDA has refused to take any action to legally prohibit the use of MSG in American baby food. In fact, the FDA has steadfastly refused to consider any research that challenges their viewpoint that MSG is a safe additive in the American food supply.

One of the main effects of MSG is to trigger a sharp increase in insulin production. This leads to fat storage and a "food craving" response. One way to test this is to make a short list of the foods you crave and then check their labels. With some research, you will find that nearly all (if not indeed every one) are MSG rich foods.

One difficulty in identifying the presence of MSG in our food is that the FDA has allowed it to be very loosely labeled in over 40 different ingredients, few of which give any clue that MSG is present. MSG is always present in the following ingredients: yeast, gelatin, whey protein, pectin, natural beef flavoring, soy protein stock, enzymes, powdered milk, broth, "seasonings", bouillon, citric acid, malt extract, "flavor" and "flavorings," and many others. MSG can even be found in salad dressings, ice creams, cheeses, medications, frozen meals, chewing gum and cigarettes.

Setting scientific studies aside for a moment, here is what we can easily and safely conclude about MSG. It makes us crave foods that have been artificially enhanced to make us eat more. It makes us fatter at the expense of more balanced natural foods that would make us thinner, healthier, and happier. All of which leads to the list of....

FOODS THAT KILL
- Hamburgers, steaks, ribs, meat loaf, pork, mutton
- sausage, bacon, spam, processed deli meats
- processed sugar & salt

- FRIED FOODS (except egg whites)
- CANNED FOODS with salt or sugar added
- MOST CHEESE & foods that contain cheese (For pizza, use soy or low fat, low sodium cheese)
- White Bread/Rolls, White Rice, White Pasta
- CEREALS with added sugar
- SALTY SNACKS (chips, pretzels, nuts, margarine, etc.)
- Butter, coffee creams (Replace butter with olive oil)
- Cake, candy, ice cream, cookies, pie, soft drinks
- Donuts, sorbet, salted nuts
- Corn & many syrups; anything artificial

> *You can't lose weight by talking about it.*
> *You have to keep your mouth shut.*
> —unknown

BRAIN HIJACKING FOODS

It's no secret. In combination, the foods above can smack your brain hard enough to make it go haywire and cause you to overeat, binge, grow fatter, get sick, and die too soon. As a nation, millions of us are doing it every day.

Even breads spike our appetites, causing us to overeat. Steak, sausage, bacon, and their meaty cousins sooner or later provoke our own hearts to attack us. Salty snack foods are bad for both brain and body.

And then there's all the sweet stuff. Try this simple test. Place a photograph of a carrot next to one of a carrot cake. Then see which photograph you focus on, the healthful one or the harmful one? Then decide for yourself how healthy is that part of your brain involved in making food choices.

If this test result motivates you to try to regain food sanity, the mere act of pursuing it could be a great beginning on the road to recover. Begin your recovery by keeping away from addictive items such as salted nuts, canned foods that contain ingredients you can't pronounce or spell (read labels!), and all the foods and their obvious cousins on the "death" list of harmful foods.

Oatmeal, shredded wheat, and some other "natural" cereals are foods that don't insult your eating intelligence by adding sugar and salt. They are tasty and satisfying, especially with raisins, bananas, blueberries, and rice or soy milk. Sugared and salted foods spike food cravings and assault your brain. You lose memory. Your immune system begins attacking phantom invaders. You eat more food and enjoy it less than thinner folks. Your brain goes haywire. You overcompensate by eating still more. You binge. You want the same harmful foods again and again, and so it goes.

Then our hearts become "the" problem. We get diabetes. We take pills that make zombies of us, or cause depression. Then comes a mini stroke or three. Then hospitalization. Then the grief and the goodbyes, and we get so tired. Then we decide to die after one of our major organs fail. Sad as all this is for those who give a damn about us, what's worse are those 10 or 15 years of needless suffering we first must endure because of all the overeating of harmful foods.

So improve your food choices and all those "health" care providers out there won't get to apply their painful, expensive "treatment" to you. Discipline yourself to eat less, but higher quality foods. Become your own number one provider of health care. Who knows more about what you need than you?

Walk a lot more. Sit a lot less. Ladies and gentlemen, it's in your hands; health or sickness, a longer, healthier life, or one shortened by a lousy lifestyle. Looking at things this way makes pork chops and peppermint patties unappealing.

> *The doctor of the future will give us no medication,*
> *but will interest his patients in the care of the human frame,*
> *diet, and in the cause and prevention of disease.*
> — Thomas Edison

WHAT TO DO

The food industry wants to keep us buying their processed foods, and they have been successful at it. We are addicted in record numbers from coast to coast, and we're becoming fatter than ever. If we want to transform ourselves, we have to also transform our minds and habits. Knowing what we now know about additives in our food supply, we have to think outside of the Devil's Food cookie box. We need to realize that our true freedom lies in buying and eating healthful natural foods whenever we can.

For our health, for our true happiness, for our freedom, and for the sakes of those who love us, we need to wake up, make and smell and enjoy some delicious homemade vegetable soup. Let a healthful revolution happen now in our own bodies.

HOW THE WORLD'S OLDEST MAN DID IT

Walter Breuning, at 113, said he lived as long as he has because he left every meal a little bit hungry and limited his meals to two per day for the past 35 years of his life. "You should push back from the table when you're still hungry."

He eats a big breakfast and lunch every day, but no supper. "I have weighed the same (135 lbs., 5'8") for 35 years, and that's about the way it should be. You get in the habit of not eating at night and you realize how good you feel . . . if you could just tell people not to eat so darn much."

Breakfast for Breuning comes before 8 a.m. and usually consists of eggs, toast, or pancakes. "I eat a lot of fruit every day."

He also takes a baby aspirin. "Just one baby aspirin, that's the only pill I ever take, no other medicine."

And he drinks lots of water. "I drink water all the time plus coffee. I drink a cup and a half of coffee for breakfast and a cup with lunch." The world's oldest man said he's been healthy his entire life and believes diet played a large part of it.

"Everybody was poor years ago. When we were kids, we ate what was on the table. Crusts of bread or whatever it was. You ate what they put on your plate, and that's all you got."

He also believes that working hard has helped extend his life. "Work never hurt anybody." Breuning's last job ended at age 99. On eating out: "Once you get used to not eating in restaurants, you don't want to anymore."

MacDonald's™ in Tokyo is a terrible revenge for Pearl Harbor.
—SI Hayakawa

IV.

Dental

Why Dentists Don't Play Basketball

*If apples keep doctors away, will dentists play
more basketball when our mouths are healthy?*
—Mike Shane

A DENTIST DOESN'T TEACH US MUCH ABOUT OUR MOUTHS FOR THE
same reason doctors don't teach much about the rest of us.
Teaching good health doesn't "make" a good (enough) income.
Patching decayed teeth and treating rotted gums makes dentists a
lot of money. Much less income would result once we learn and
practice good dental hygiene.

So if we really want to live with healthy teeth and gums in
our mouths, we better learn, on our own, to care properly for
ourselves.

A typical dentist or his/her assistant usually says a few things:
Floss more, brush better, and cut down on the sweet stuff. This

sounds OK but is simply babble in terms of helpfulness. We haven't learned HOW to prevent the diseases and problems that visit our mouths whether it's gums that bleed or teeth that, in their wisdom, hurt. A healthy mouth needs no x-rays, periodic cleanings, fillings, dentures, root canals, gold crowns, etc. Why haven't we been taught (until now) or learned how to keep our mouths healthy?

> *The first thing I do in the morning is brush*
> *my teeth and sharpen my tongue.*
> —Dorothy Parker

Here's a "do you know" quiz on whether you properly care for your mouth, gums, and teeth.

Do you use a dental water jet? If not, you aren't doing enough for your gums. What about a soft bristle toothbrush? If you brush with hard bristles, tooth enamel can wear down. Not using dental floss daily? That'll eventually become a pain to both mouth and wallet. Knowing how to keep your mouth clean is as good as knowing when to keep it shut. Keeping it clean will save your teeth, produce healthy gums, fatten your wallet, and extend your life.

> *Some tortures are physical and some are mental,*
> *but the one that is both is dental.*
> —Ogden Nash

Taking good dental care of yourself, like proper eating, takes some time to do correctly, but isn't difficult or THAT time consuming once you get the hang of it. Keeping your mouth and teeth healthy does require the same mindfulness that is needed to eat healthfully.

WHAT TO DO!

- *Have your teeth fixed and cleaned professionally one final time, preferably at a dental school because it's free. That becomes your baseline.*

Guidelines that follow should keep your teeth healthy and your gums free of further disease from then on.

> *If a patient cannot clean his teeth, no*
> *dentist can clean them for him.*
> —Martin H. Fischer

NIGHT FLOSSING IS THE RIGHT FLOSSING

- FLOSS every night before bedtime to maintain healthy teeth and gums. Flossing AND using a water jet help provide maximum removal of decay causing bacteria. These bacterial devils multiply 30 times overnight in our mouths when allowed to lie around and make unbothered love. Both flossing and using a Waterpik™ are necessary for our victories in bacterial warfare. They help each other achieve the best outcome.

- UN-WAXED dental floss is best for most of us. Waxed dental floss can seal food particles further into gums, which is opposite of what we want. The main purpose of flossing is to scrape plaque off teeth and extract food particles from underneath gums and between teeth.

- Oral B™ brand "ultra" dental floss works well. Unlike ordinary floss, it's made out of spongy nylon fibers that stretch thin to fit easily into tight spaces between teeth. Then the fibers spring back to the original thickness to "flick away" plaque. Inexpensive UN-WAXED floss sold at groceries and pharmacies works OK. Remember, the main purpose of flossing is to SCRAPE OFF plaque attached to teeth or pull out small food particles that have been hiding between teeth and/or under gums since you last chewed something.

FLOSSING CORRECTLY: Guide dental floss between your teeth using a gentle rubbing motion against the sides. Don't snap the floss into your gums. When the floss reaches the gum line, gently slide it into the space between the gum and tooth and flick it upward. Hold the floss tightly against the tooth, rubbing it from the gum with upward motions. Learn as much as you can about plaque and tartar and why your teeth decay, and your gums get sick. Daily flossing is essential to the health of your mouth, and to the rest of you.

Floss EVERY NIGHT after you finish eating. Floss during the day whenever you feel the need. When not removed, plaque turns into tartar, and tartar turns into gum disease. Diseased gums promote heart disease and strokes. Cut those connections by flossing before bedtime.

People who floss daily live longer than those who don't. Studies have found that men with gum disease have a whopping 70% higher risk of developing heart disease.

Finally, our breath improves after flossing, thereby enhancing the chances for more kissing, cuddling, and fooling around.

> *A man loses his illusions first, his teeth*
> *second, his follies last.*
> —Helen Rowland

Hate to Floss?

If you simply WON'T floss even after we scared you half to death, here's another option: Thin toothpicks. Like floss, toothpicks clean around the gum area and between teeth and are easy to use. Try Doctor's Brush picks™ (our favorite by far). It works with your water jet to remove food particles that cause gum and teeth problems.

For best results, use all the dental aids mentioned in this section: water jet, un-waxed floss, toothpicks, electric toothbrush, etc. Using them will get your teeth and gums looking and feeling their best. All by yourself, you can prevent gum disease and tooth decay from now on. Yes you can.

> *She laughs at everything you say. Why?*
> *Because she has fine teeth.*
> —Benjamin Franklin

WATER JETTING

Water jets are the most helpful dental devices hardly anyone knows much about. If you live with teeth and gums in your mouth, using a water jet is at least as important as brushing and flossing every day. Why on God's earth, we wonder, has professional dentistry done so little to educate us about the terrific dental benefits of a water jet? Use it daily and your gums probably won't bleed anymore and will look and feel healthier too. Dangerous gingivitis is likely to leave you alone.

A water jet works safely, fast, and effectively to force food particles harboring bacteria out from between our teeth and from below the gum line. When you combine the benefits of a water jet with flossing and healthful eating, your gums and teeth will remain as healthy as nature intended before sugary foods started dominating our diets.

Sadly, nearly 80% of adult Americans don't floss (or use a water jet during teeth cleaning). About 20% say it takes too much time. Another 25% say they either forget or are too lazy to floss. So dental disease is now a national epidemic, like obesity. But we CAN join those 20% of dental winners who floss properly to protect their oral health.

Corporate Mischief

Do not be misled by the water jet folks who want you to believe their product works "better" than dental floss. These two dental aids do overlap to some extent in terms of how they clean your mouth, but they emphasize different aspects of the cleaning process. They complement each other. Better outcomes happen when both are used rather than one or the other. Check out their respective benefits.

If you intend to keep your teeth free of decay, you need to floss every night and use the water jet after meals and snacks. Use the money you save on dental bills for extra Florida vacations, or buying more "Victory" diet books to give your friends and family. Dental health is good for everyone.

Water jets massage and strengthen your gums, improving blood circulation. This halts bleeding. The jets work by delivering water at a high pressure of a thousand or more pulses per minute.

The combination of water pressure and pulsation removes debris and bacteria hiding between teeth and below the gum line.

After meals, use the jets. Waterpik™ is a popular brand. Combine flossing and jetting and toothpicks and your teeth and gums will live healthfully as long as the rest of you. Not bad for an electric dental tool that costs less than 50 bucks and is sold at thousands of stores.

> *I told my dentist my teeth were going yellow.*
> *He told me to wear a brown tie.*
> —Rodney Dangerfield

Benefits of Water Jetting

- Gums get massaged and stimulated. Gum health is restored. Bleeding stops. Jetting gets finished fast.
- Food particles and bacteria hiding between teeth and below the gum line are removed safely. Gum disease is prevented.
- Our breath freshens.
- If invited, a portable water jet will go to work with you.
- WARM water and/or mouthwash may be used in any combination.
- Braces, etc. are not disturbed by a water jet.

Brushing Your Teeth

> *You don't have to brush your teeth,*
> *just the ones you want to keep.*
> —unknown

What matters is for you to brush your teeth the right way at least twice a day, after breakfast and before you go to sleep. Proper brushing, along with flossing, water jetting, and eating health-fully are why your teeth and gums will remain disease free from now on.

Keep an extra toothbrush/toothpaste in a handy place at work next to your portable water jet. This makes them easy to use after lunch, or snacks (nuts, crackers, raisins, etc.).

The "right" toothbrush should contain SOFT nylon bristles with round ends. Medium and hard bristles can be abrasive and wear down teeth. The ORAL B™ brand toothbrush is a good idea because the company ONLY sells soft bristle brushes.

COLGATE™ TOOTHPASTE

Wet the brush slightly and squeeze a small amount of toothpaste onto it. Colgate Total Clean Mint toothpaste contains fluoride and leaves a fresh taste in the mouth. Colgate says this tooth-paste prevents cavities, gingivitis, plaque, and fights tartar build-up. Giant companies like Colgate have to tell the truth, don't they? In any event, Total Clean Mint is a good paste.

Brush away from your gums to clean the outside and inside surfaces of the teeth. Use short strokes. Brush gently along the gum line. Gum disease begins here so you want to get it clean but avoid damaging your gums. Brush your tongue, the roof of your mouth, and your cheeky sides. All may harbor bacteria that needs to be removed.

Slosh some water around your mouth, then spit it into the sink. Your brushing is complete and your mouth now feels good.

ELECTRIC TOOTHBRUSH

Why use a manual toothbrush? A power toothbrush with "ro-tation oscillation" gets your teeth and gums a lot cleaner a lot quicker. Buy yourself one like the Oral B™ Vitality toothbrush for about 20 bucks. You'll be glad you did.

NIGHT-TIME DENTAL HYGIENE PERFECTION

- Use a water jet to dislodge, remove most food particles.
  —2 minutes

- Use floss (and/or toothpick) to scrape plaque from teeth, and from under gum line. —4 minutes

- Use water jet (again) to remove plaque loosened but left behind by the dental floss. —1 minute

- Brush your teeth to polish them, and clean the tongue and roof of your mouth. —2 minutes

The devil fears the Word of God, but can't bite it.
It breaks his teeth.
—Martin Luther

V.

Day & Night Exercises

AFTER IMPROVING YOUR FOOD CHOICES, EXERCISE IS THE SECOND key to a new you. When it becomes a daily event, exercising can be a big winner for dieters. Find an exercise you can do twice daily for at least 30–45 minutes per session and it will be make you healthier and thinner. You can mix and match exercises and can break sessions into as many as you like to achieve your overall minutes target, and that's what's important. Within a few weeks, you'll feel healthy results inside and you will see them on the outside.

Feeling great on the inside is good, but many dieters exercise to look great on the outside. Think of exercise as a safe medicine that can improve your opinion of yourself. Once you put it to that test, you will find that exercising is far better than anything you can buy at the drugstore, or find in your medicine cabinet.

However, if exercising were easy, everyone would have perfect bodies. If eating right and exercising were simple, heart disease would not be the nation's number one death maker. The fact is that starting an exercise program is unpleasant and difficult. Celebrities do not maintain their thin appearance because they love to exercise. They pay millions every year for fitness professionals to motivate them. Whether you are famous or infamous, the hardest part about exercising is generating the motivation to stick with it. What you need for successful exercising are secrets that offer you staying power. These are the power of Why.

The only exercise some people get is jumping to conclusions,
running down their friends, side-stepping responsibility,
and pushing their luck!
—unknown

THE POWER OF WHY

Let's say you are walking along the beach and you find a bottle in the sand. Let's say a genie appeared out of the bottle and offers you the best 2 for 1 deal you can imagine. Two hours would be added to your life for every hour of exercise you complete. As much as you hate to exercise, would you refuse?

Well, the genie's deal is for real. According to the American Heart Association, you can take advantage of this magical 2 for 1 deal anytime—no beach and no genie required. But it doesn't just stop at adding years onto your life. In this deal, you also will receive a higher quality of life attached to your remaining years. Think of it as Mother Nature's 401k plan for your life. For every hour of exercise, she not only gives you matching funds, but doubles them. And then she sweetens the deal. You get a better life with fewer hospital stays, less stress for your family, and more enjoyment for you.

My idea of exercise is a good brisk sit.
—Phyllis Diller

What's the use of living longer if we can't be there for the ones we love? Exercise is the remedy for not only living longer, but living better with an improved mental outlook, a more enjoyable sex life at any age, and being there for our loved ones with a healthy mind/body, and not being a burden.

We all want to enjoy life. The trick is finding the right kind of joy. We're out of shape from enjoying life in the wrong ways. But there is hope for us. Instead of feeling like we will die from giving up the "joy" of eating harmful things and a lifestyle of comfort food and sofa time, we can rejoice at improving our lives by eating more deliciously and nutritionally, and exercising. We will live smarter, not harder.

Think about it this way; a longer healthy productive life, with more joy, or a shorter life with more disease. When we think of choices this way, the temporary discomfort of beginning an exercise program begins to look OK. Don't think of it in terms of whether you have time to exercise. Instead, think of it in terms of how much your loved ones will miss you if you don't.

> *Being entirely honest with oneself is a good exercise.*
> —Sigmund Freud

Here's your choice. Exercise every day or get sick and need a heart bypass operation at some stage, and have a medical somebody you don't know (more importantly, who doesn't know you) cut you up. Assuming you recover from the operation, guess what you will be told after leaving the hospital and filling your new prescriptions? . . . that you need to begin an exercise program. So you can start exercising should you survive a heart attack, or you can start now. You are an intelligent person. Start now and to hell with excuses.

REASONS TO EXERCISE

* A third of American adults have some sort of cardiac problem. About 16 percent of men between 20 and 39 have at least one symptom and eight percent of women. About 38 percent

of men and women between 40 and 59 have heart problems. The rates skyrocket to 73 percent after the age of 60.

- Obesity can reduce your lifespan by 20 years. Even if you are just overweight and not obese, your lifespan will be shorter.

- You are not alone. Six out of 10 Americans are overweight or obese. But who wants to be a member of the society of fatness? Not you, or you wouldn't still be reading this book. In addition to weight control, exercise helps prevent or reverse heart disease. It helps control cholesterol levels and diabetes. It slows bone loss associated with advancing age, lowers the risk of certain cancers, and helps reduce anxiety.

- Fewer than one in three Americans exercise regularly at recommended levels, and nearly two-thirds of them are overweight or obese. See the connection here?

- A difference of one can of soda a day (150 calories) or 60 minutes of brisk daily walking can add OR subtract over 15 pounds to your weight each year. Just imagine if you eliminated pop AND decided to walk about an hour a day. You would double your results and lose 30 pounds in a year. Knowing this, can you really ever say again with a straight face that Coke™ is it?

- Think of exercise as food to realize what you are burning off. One hour of walking burns off the calorie equivalent of a typical jelly filled doughnut (300 calories). You can also do the reverse and think of food as exercise. Before you stop at the drive-thru on your way home from work, consider that a double-cheeseburger with large fries and a 24 ounce soft drink (1500 calories) is equivalent to 2.5 hours of running at a 10 minute per mile pace.

> *Fitness—if it came in a bottle, everybody would*
> *have a great body.*
> —Cher

Now, if you are committed to losing weight and getting in better shape, which is easier—driving past the drive-thru and going home for a nutritious vegetable soup, or running 2.5 hours? Put it this way: I haven't seen any restaurant make a double cheeseburger that anyone should run after for even five minutes, let alone for over two hours. Exercising is essential to weight loss and you need to learn enough about it (books, gyms, Internet) to determine which mix of the many splendid exercises (swimming, jogging, biking, hiking, gardening, yoga, weight training, etc.) will serve you best. This book will focus on just two helpful exercises: Walking: the easiest; and sex, the one that's fun.

> *Another good reducing exercise consists in*
> *placing both hands against the table edge and pushing back.*
> —Robert Quillen

WALK BRISKLY OR DON'T BOTHER

Walk for at least an hour a day. Walk as if you need to get somewhere else fast, at least as far away as possible from your refrigerator. The number of daily walks you take doesn't matter, it's the total daily walking time that counts. Once walking becomes routine and easy for you, mix some slow jogging into your walk, especially down hills. This will get your heart pumping, providing additional benefits.

Besides helping you lose weight, walking briskly once or twice a day adds to your overall well being. Here are some reasons to stop reading this book for awhile and take a walk:

- Walking is good for the brain. Women who walk a lot have better brain function than those who walk less.

- Walking is good for bones. Walkers have higher leg bone density than non-walkers.

- Walking strengthens the heart and cuts the risk of heart attack. Walkers live longer than non-walkers.

- Walking mindfully can help remove mental clutter and chatter that we carry with us. That's especially so when we walk in a nice area, mindful of the pleasant surroundings.

> *Anywhere is walking distance if you've got the time.*
> —Stephen Wright

- While you walk, count the trees or bushes that pass you by, or the steps you take, or the breaths you make. When you get home, you will feel better. Sit down to enjoy a cup of peppermint tea and continue reading this book.
- Daily walks improve heart and lung fitness. Your entire body will work better. Walking with a friend makes the experience more enjoyable. Time goes by faster when you're talking some talk while walking the walk. Still, walking alone is better than not walking at all.

> *Walking with a friend in the dark is better*
> *than walking alone in the light.*
> —Helen Keller

Everyone knows that brisk walking for an hour or more every day is great for the legs, heart, butt, and other parts, but did you know that a daily walk can help flatten your belly? After 14 weeks of brisk walking, women in one study shrunk belly fat by 20 percent, without cutting back their eating.

When we dedicate an hour or more a day to walking, we increase the possibility that three of life's major goals can be achieved—a longer life, fewer illnesses, and less weight. The longer the walks, the lower the weight, the better your health.

Walking is a low stress, low sweat answer to lifetime conditioning. Don't forget to swing your arms as you walk. They don't want to be left behind swinging in the breeze.

> *A vigorous five mile walk will do more good than*
> *all the medicine and psychology in the world.*
> —Dr. Carl Dudley White

BEDROOM OLYMPICS

Walking every day and less eating may revive the dormant sex drive of obese men. It reversed impotence (albeit after two years) in about a third of obese men with erectile dysfunction. Exercising plus better diet is credited with making a positive difference for men in the bedroom. Men who exercise engage in sex ten years longer than men who don't.

> *I consider exercise vulgar. It makes people smell.*
> —Alec Thornton

When you have lots of sex, you lose weight. When you lose weight, the sex gets better. Being overweight affects your sex drive, but small changes can jump-start your appetite for lovemaking. Sex helps you lose weight because it produces feel-good hemicals in the brain. They are so satisfying that your brain forgets to send you other signals, like the one directing you to raid the refrigerator.

Because being overweight and being sexy do not mix, here's what you can do to restore yourself to exciting sexual days of yesteryear:

- Lose weight. As little as 10 pounds can stimulate sex hormones.
- Replace harmful foods with more nutritious foods.
- Some of your workout exercises should be designed to generate blood flow to the pelvic area.
- Read a sex or sexy novel. Watch some porn. Activate the erotic section of your mind.
- Believe you have become a very sexy person and prove it by renewing intimacy with someone special.

> *Don't have sex man. It leads to kissing and pretty*
> *soon you have to start talking to them.*
> —Steve Martin

Exercising in bed is a great way to lose weight and get fit, according to one expert (a housewife). "I recommend having sex about five times a week. Since it's free and a lot of fun, making love is my favorite form of exercise."

Sex becomes an exercise when you move about, on, under and beside your partner either face to face, or top to bottom. If you're an overweight man and it hasn't been getting up, use another part to please her/him. Unlike a lazy penis, the tip of the tongue is usually willing to obey bedroom instructions. It can delight even the most reluctant of play partners.

Remember, what you give in bed is what's likely coming back to you. Become creatively playful and not boringly automatic. Play the role of the self assured lover your bed partner has always yearned for. Good sex is about intimacy—physical and emotional intimacy, and yes, even conversational intimacy. Mental lovemaking counts even more than the right touch. So say something loving and sexy, and mean it. You know what she/he wants you to say. You have already walked the walk, so now it's time to talk the (right) talk.

Good sex is about friends getting together and pleasing each other in enjoyably imaginative ways. Otherwise, what's the point?

Too many of us receive or offer too little emotional and physical love so we try to compensate by overeating. Without the touch of a loved one, we poke around the refrigerator trying to find some THING satisfying to eat, to replace some one to love.

Love and love-making therefore can be about becoming thinner. When you get thinner, the sex gets better. When the sex is good, you want more of it, and probably less food. Why? Because we want to have more energy for more sex, and eating too much tires us out.

> *I'm at the age when food has taken the place of*
> *sex in my life. In fact, I've just had a mirror*
> *put over my kitchen table.*
> —Rodney Dangerfield

Becoming thinner also means that being overweight is no longer embarrassing. As you get thinner, you'll want sex more often. If you are in a relationship, it will become more loving. If not, begin looking for someone out there to love. The point is to replace the "what's for dinner" chatter with "let's skip dinner so we can play".

> *My love life is terrible. The last time I was*
> *inside a woman was when I visited the Statue of Liberty.*
> —Woody Allen

If you do enough of it, sex can help make you thinner. Interest your partner in the "new sexual you" and you both could fall in love all over again. Nearly all of us love to be touched in both therapeutic and sensual ways. ALL of us want to be loved, and to be in love. Replacing weight with love is a good exchange. Five sex sessions a week averaging about 30 minutes can burn over 1,000 calories. That's good poundage off your butt in just a few weeks.

Before sex, shower together, exchange massages, and other warm-ups. Make sure the warm-up to sex is wonderful. Perhaps sip some wine. Not only will the love-making become much better, but your partner will want to hang out with you more because you're a lot of fun. You're more loving, and more beloved in lots of ways.

Benefits of quality sex include:

- Less body fat
- Better muscle tone
- Improved blood circulation
- Better sleep
- More energy
- Decreased stress
- Improved life overall

> *When I'm good, I'm very, very good,*
> *but when I'm bad I'm better.*
> —Mae West

Sexually active women produce more estrogen. Hair is shinier. Thanks to sweating, skin pores are cleansed. Both sexes feel and look younger from frequent sex. We are happier, better rested, and more content with our lives.

Putting passion into love-making makes it become more fun and frequent. Engaging in satisfying sex leads to the desire for even more, and it becomes a healthful cycle that, like walking, feeds upon itself. It takes our minds out of the refrigerator.

But be sure your health can hold up under the (positive) stress of more vigorous sex. What you want are loving, passionate bedroom romps, not a quick trip to the emergency room or cardiac care unit of some hospital. Before you jump into bedroom Olympic events with nothing but naughtiness on your mind, get into decent shape, perhaps even visit a medical somebody.

> *It's not true I had nothing on. I had the radio on.*
> —Marilyn Monroe

VI.
Path to a Miracle, Part 2

For me the sunshine state had become God's waiting room. Three loving relatives flew in to pack, load, and deliver me to a small apartment on a hilltop near Charlottesville, home of the University of Virginia. That was the summer of 2006 and good things soon began to happen.

> *Miracles happen to those who believe in them.*
> —Bernard Berenson

No longer was dying me dwelling in a Valley of the Shadow of Death trading medical horror stories with dying neighbors. Even if Uncle Jerry found me hiding on that hill, at least a pretty student nurse may be holding my hand when I had to board his bus.

My arm returned from the dead on its own. I spoke again although the words came slowly, much too slowly, formulated by an obviously injured brain. I limped around for more months, a visual statement to all that I was a sick man. But in Virginia, at least for now, Uncle Jerry left me alone. Except for one "nationally renown expert" at the University of Virginia, doctors didn't push operations. I took three medicines daily; aspirin (made from a tree), Digoxin™ (from a plant growing in backyards), and a water pill. None produced discernable side effects.

If your time hasn't come, even a doctor can't kill you.
—MA Perlstein

The first week in Virginia I walked downtown looking for the state wine store. Instead a tiny medical shop on Main Street drew my attention. It looked like it came right out of an episode of the Twilight Zone. Perhaps 50 serious illnesses were listed (or rather plastered) on the storefront window; problems that could be treated inside. These included heart disease and stroke, so I opened the door.

"Come in. I can help you." Dr. Q (PhD) was standing alone. He reminded me of Pat Morita, the Mr. Miyagi character in the Karate Kid. His was a kindly face with a confident body posture. I asked him to sell me some medicines (observable on the shelf).

"It doesn't work that way. First you need to be my patient. I find out what's wrong, then you can buy medicine." Being Dr. Q's patient cost $100 for a comprehensive first exam/treatment (2 hours), and $50 for each visit (one hour) afterwards. He was "retired" and opened the office to treat one or two patients a day to have something to do away from home, and because "work is good". Money wasn't his motivator.

Before "retirement" to Charlottesville, Dr. Q taught physicians in Japan how to heal patients without harming them.

If you realize that all things change, there is nothing
you will try to hold onto. If you are not afraid of
dying, there is nothing you cannot achieve.
—unknown

The dozens of doctors I met over a lifetime carried a medical kit containing three or four tools designed to help their patients get better (prescriptions, surgery, advice). Dr. Q's medical toolbox must've contained 30 more. Special menus were offered to feed my sick heart because "the right food is your best medicine". Acupuncture needles darted into my ear lobes and other places without bloodshed. He literally smashed into smithereens "knots" in my upper back that didn't belong there. Herbs were formulated into medicines and capsulated by him at the office during the appointment. He taught stand-still workout routines that allowed my body to watch TV while being exercised. There was music or chanting that promoted healing. Some treatment techniques were so awesome, I tended not to believe, even as the paranormal stuff was being applied on me. So I won't pursue that EXCEPT for the miracle(s) Dr. Q predicted and showed me how to make happen.

All in all, this man from Asia, in "retirement", made conventional American medical practice seem comparatively pathetic. At the end of the fifth session, he summarized my medical situation.

"Mr. Shane, you're very sick, and I can't save you." (Not a big surprise)

"What now?"

"Find someone to love you, to take care of you. SHE will save your life."

Where there is great love, there are always miracles.
—Willa Cather

"No sir. THAT won't happen. A woman's never taken care of me before, or loved me all that much for that matter. (Some didn't have time for it.)

Stupid me. I was arguing with a wise, wonderful man.

"Dr. Q, I just moved here. I don't know any woman who would love me. I can't even get it up anymore. Why bother?"

> *There are four questions of value in life.*
> *What is sacred? Of what is the Spirit made?*
> *What is worth living for and what is worth dying for?*
> *The answer to each is the same, only love.*
> —Don Juan deMarco

Dr. Q persevered. "Ask your relatives to help. They'll help you find someone."

"They don't live here, Dr. Q. Anyway, the ones who would do it, are dead."

"Who's your favorite relative?"

"Grandma Gussie. She died over 25 years ago."

"No, she's with you. She wants to help. Go home and ask her to help you."

I talked to Grandma Gussie that night. (How could it hurt?)

"Grandma, it's me, Michael. First of all, I love you. I miss you. (Tears filled my eyes for the first time in decades.) I apologize for not talking to you until now. Never thought to do it, and I'm sorry for asking you for a favor so soon. My doctor says you will help me find a woman to love me and to save my life, perhaps someone wonderful like you, Grandma? (finally I was getting smart). I know you are happy in heaven. Give my love to Betty (my mother), and Suzie and Rozie (younger sisters).

> *There are two ways to live your life. One is as though nothing*
> *ever is a miracle. The other is as though everything is a miracle.*
> —Albert Einstein

Dear reader: It's no surprise to you and no miracle that The NEXT day I found someone special and smart (PhD), who saved my life. But that wonderful event COULD have been a very lucky break, and no miracle. It could have been something like winning some lottery, and lots of people do that.

We sipped coffee downtown and were living together a week later. (This is supposed to be a diet/health enhancement book, not a romance novel, so relationship details are for the next book. What carried an extraordinarily lucky and wonderful event out of the realm of good luck and into the paranormal and world of miracles, is this: The love of my life looked EXACTLY like Grandma Gussie when both were 47 years young. In my view, THAT cannot be explained away as a coincidence.

My health was OK during the first year of our relationship. Then the love of my life saved my life, just as Doctor Q said she would.

> *I am a realist. I expect miracles.*
> —Wayne Dyer

Here's what happened. Before striking, all three strokes provided the same specific warning signals; pain in my limbs and upper back. When those pains came again in 2007, I knew what to expect. Stroke number 4 was on the way.

I told my love to pack up and return to the home she still owned. She ought not be part of some dreadful stroke scene. She was silent for half an hour, then said what would save my life, and liberate me from strokes since then.

"I don't want to leave, but before you kick me out, try one more thing. Your food choices contain too much salt. Cut back on salty foods and let's see what happens."

I did. Two days later I was pain free and have remained so. Nobody before my darling so pointedly and clearly shared how my mindless eating of salty foods could lead to strokes.

Summarizing: Miracle one was Grandma Gussie finding me the right woman. Dr. Q's prediction that this lovely person would save my life was, in my view, the second miracle.

What can we take from this? Well, perhaps our favorite grandma can make miracles happen, and we should ask her when we need one (or ANY other relative who loves us). It worked for cynical, skeptical, non-believing me. Since then, I have lived years longer than anyone, including me, thought possible; long enough and healthy enough to write this book. Could similar miracles happen for you? Why not!

> *For three days after death, hair and fingernails*
> *continue to grow, but phone calls taper off.*
> —Johnny Carson

Anyway, here I am. It's Feb. 15, 2010, and Uncle Jerry may be out there somewhere looking for me or peddling salt for that matter, but I don't care. I am comforted by miracles and Grandma Gussie, and the love of my life, and by the remarkable Dr. Q.

Now YOU know how miracles can happen. Make one happen for you!

> *And in the end, the love you take is*
> *equal to the love you make.*
> —Sir Paul McCartney

If you have questions, comments, or if you want a discount on additional books for friends and family, email Shane: Moshe4442003@yahoo.com.